AN INTRODUCTION
TO CLINICAL
RHEUMATOLOGY

The Author

WILLIAM CARSON DICK
M.D.(Glasgow), M.R.C.P.(Lond.)

Arthritis and Rheumatism Council Lecturer in Medicine,
University Department of Medicine,
Royal Infirmary, Glasgow, and
Centre for Rheumatic Diseases, Glasgow

An Introduction to Clinical Rheumatology

WILLIAM CARSON DICK

CHURCHILL LIVINGSTONE
EDINBURGH LONDON AND NEW YORK
1972

CHURCHILL LIVINGSTONE

Medical Division of Longman Group Limited

Distributed in the United States of America by
Churchill Livingstone Inc., 19 West 44th Street, New York,
N.Y. 10036 and by associated companies,
branches and representatives throughout
the world.

First published 1972
Reprinted   1977
Reprinted   1978
Reprinted   1979

ISBN 0 443 00762 4

Printed in Hong Kong by Wah Cheong Printing Press Ltd

FOREWORD

The conditions which comprise what is now accepted as the sub-speciality of rheumatology have rarely received from clinicians and educators the interest and attention that their frequency and morbidity merit. Their clinical course is more likely to be disabling than dramatic, their pathogenesis is still often ill understood, and their management is in consequence usually empirical rather than specific. Dr Dick has, within a brief compass, written an up-to-date and practical account of the essentials of rheumatology which should be helpful to senior medical students and interested physicians.

Department of Medicine,
University of Glasgow, 1972

EDWARD M. McGIRR

PREFACE

This introductory textbook on the rheumatic diseases is based upon lectures given to undergraduate medical students at Glasgow University and to postgraduate practitioners at the Royal College of Physicians and Surgeons, Glasgow. It is my hope that the book contains sufficient information for postgraduates preparing for the M.R.C.P. examination and yet is concise enough for the interested undergraduate.

I wish to thank Professor E. M. McGirr, Professor W. Watson Buchanan and all my colleagues at the Centre for Rheumatic Diseases for their help and encouragement. I would also like to express my appreciation to Brenda Burn at the Royal Infirmary, Glasgow, who prepared the figures, Mrs M. Skene, who typed the manuscript.

1972   W. CARSON DICK

CONTENTS

Chapter 1

INTRODUCTION

'Rheumatic diseases are fast becoming Western Europe's most prevalent, most expensive and most neglected group of diseases.' (W.H.O., 1962)

This rather startling statement by an otherwise somewhat conservative body highlights the growing awareness of the medical, social and economic burden which the rheumatic diseases impose upon highly developed countries. In a recent United Kingdom survey rheumatic complaints were found to be second only to accidents in the numbers affected and second only to bronchitis in the number of working days lost. Arthritis and rheumatism accounted for 11 per cent of the total number of working days lost from all causes, the annual cost to the nation being approximately £190 million.

From the point of view of the family doctor complaints due to arthritis and rheumatism were the leading cause of consultations in female patients and were exceeded only by respiratory complaints in males.

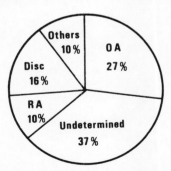

Fig. 1 Relative prevalence of the arthritides in the population. OA. osteo-arthrosis; RA, rheumatoid arthritis.

It is essential to appreciate the overall prevalence of the individual members of the rheumatic diseases. As can be seen in Figure 1 nearly 40 per cent of rheumatic complaints are of undetermined aetiology. This presents a challenge to all practitioners working in this field. A great deal of work remains to be done in this area to provide information which will contribute to our understanding of the pathogenesis of these diseases. Although this group of rheumatic complaints is so common our ignorance of it is almost total and therefore no chapter is devoted to this subject.

The second most common of the rheumatic diseases is osteoarthrosis, accounting for 27 per cent of the total, and degenerative disc disease follows at 16 per cent. Rheumatoid arthritis is less common than osteoarthrosis but accounts for a greater amount of disability. The sum of all of the seronegative arthritides and the connective tissue diseases make up only 10 per cent of the total.

Chapter 2

THE NORMAL JOINT

Joints which possess a synovial lined cavity are called diarthrodial joints and those without a joint cavity are termed synarthroses.

The diarthrodial joints differ widely in structure and function but all possess certain characteristic features (Fig. 2). Cartilage covers the expanded articulating surface of the bone and merges at its free edges with the internal synovial membrane lining of the joint cavity. Outside the synovial membrane the external lining layer of fibrous connective tissue is reinforced by the insertion of tendons and ligaments. The joint cavity contains a small amount of synovial fluid.

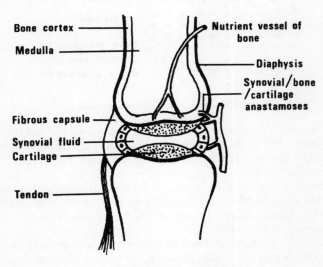

Fig. 2 The normal joint.

The cancellous bone of the diaphysis gives way to dense compact subchondral bone with few Haversian systems immediately beneath the articular surface, and this is pierced by many small blood vessel channels which loop up into the deeper areas of cartilage and also anastamose with the synovial membrane microvasculature at the synovial–cartilage junction.

Cartilage

Articular cartilage is 2 to 4 mm in thickness and is divided histologically into four layers (Fig. 3): the superficial 'tangential' zone with flattened cells; the transitional zone with large oval cells; the thick radiate zone in which the cells are arranged in radial columns; and the deep calcified zone, separated from the others by a wavy basophilic line. The three superficial zones are avascular and have no nerve fibres. The cells of articular cartilage are called chondrocytes.

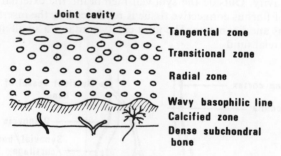

Fig. 3 Histology of cartilage (diagrammatic).

Chondrocytes possess both aerobic and anaerobic metabolic enzymes, and it is these cells which manufacture collagen. Collagen consists of fibrils of varying diameter with transverse striations, possessing a periodicity of 640Å. The biochemical hallmark of this fibrous protein is its high hydroxyproline and glycine content. Mature collagen fibres are formed from soluble fibrillar tropocollagen precursor fibres manufactured on the ribosomes of the cells.

Reticulin is closely related to collagen occurring particularly in loose connective tissue, showing the typical crossbanding of collagen fibres, and being distinguishable only by its greater affinity for silver. Elastic fibres, found in ligaments and in some fibrous capsules, consist of very fine intertwined fibrils which are not transversely striated and have a low hydroxyproline content.

The arrangement of collagen fibres in articular cartilage is currently being investigated. The old concept of a dome-shaped arrangement in accordance with lines of force has not been borne out by experimental evidence. Currently it is thought that fibres are arranged in different directions in each layer. Macroscopically the surface of articular cartilage is punctuated by irregular pits which are shown most clearly by scanning electron microscopy.

In addition to water and collagen, cartilage ground substance contains electrolytes, sialic acid and a high proportion of glycosaminoglycans, mainly chondroitin 4- and 6-sulphate, keratosulphate and some hyaluronic acid which is non-sulphated. These glycosaminoglycans are covalently bound to non-collagenous protein moieties in the matrix. Their biosynthetic pathway with the sites of involvement of insulin, thyroxine and cortisol is abbreviated in Figure 4. Whereas collagen donates strength to cartilage, the glycosaminoglycans are responsible for its elasticity by virtue of their large polyvalent molecular configurations and they are probably of importance in determining the permeability of cartilage to ionized substances.

In addition to participating in the formation of both collagen

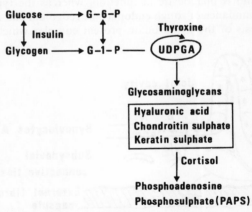

Fig. 4 Hormonal interactions with the biosynthetic pathway of the glycosaminoglycans.

and ground substance, chondrocytes possess cytoplasmic vacuoles called lysosomes. The release of destructive enzymes from these lysosomes may be implicated in disease, and consequently a great deal of research interest has centred on the stability of the lysosomal membrane and the factors which modify this. Stability of this membrane is favoured by hydrocortisone and some other anti-inflammatory drugs and prejudiced by excess vitamin A, hypoxia and bacterial infection.

Cartilage probably derives nutrition from synovial fluid by a sponge-like action. The alternate development of negative pressures in the joint at rest, and positive pressures on exercise probably plays a part in this action. The deep layer and the cartilage–synovial junction are also supplied by neighbouring blood vessels. The capacity for repair of damaged cartilage is not great although complete repair may occur.

Synovial Membrane

The synovial membrane is a complex tissue which also occurs in the lining of tendon sheaths and bursae (Fig. 4). All of the intra-articular surfaces, except the articular cartilage and some discs or menisci, are lined by a one- or two-cell thick layer of synoviocytes which is fronded in some areas. These cells are of two main types: the type A cell has numerous pinocytotic vesicles and is phagocytic in function, whereas the type B cell has an abundance of rough endoplasmic reticulum and is the site of synthesis of the hyaluronate–protein complex which confers

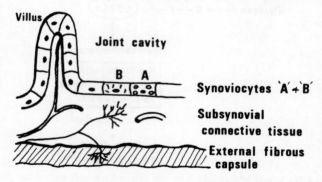

Fig. 5 Internal and external synovial membrane.

viscous properties upon synovial fluid. Many cells are inter-mediate in their characteristics.

Immediately beneath this cellular lining is the underlying connective tissue which may be areolar, adipose or fibrous in different parts of the joint and through which course the synovial blood and lymphatic vessels. Synovial fronds, or villi, are lined by synoviocytes and a central leash of blood vessels runs almost to the tip of the frond. There are very few nerve fibres in the synovial membrane.

Deep to the synovial membrane lies the fibrous capsule, or external lining, of the joint into which are inserted tendons and ligaments. This is a dense, white connective tissue layer com-posed mainly of collagen, with blood vessels and nerves running through it. Clinically this area is of significance for two reasons. Firstly, since there are so few nerve fibres in synovium or in cartilage, it seems likely that most of the pain felt in diseased joints arises either from the fibrous capsule or in exposed sub-chondral bone. Secondly, it is changes in this fibrous capsule which causes the early morning stiffness in rheumatoid arthritis.

Synovial Fluid

Normal synovial fluid is clear, viscid and weakly alkaline and is present in very small amounts. Usually less than 0.5 ml is present in the human knee, and consequently a great deal of the data presented on 'normal' synovial fluid was either obtained in animal studies or in pooled human synovial fluid samples, neither method being entirely satisfactory. It is currently rather naively assumed that synovial fluid is simply a dialysate of plasma, which is in a state of Donnan equilibrium with plasma, to which the hyaluronate–protein complex is added. The glucose level of the normal synovial fluid is less than that of serum, but the urea concentrations of blood and synovial fluid are similar. For large molecules there is a molecular weight dependent effect. Albumin is present in relatively higher concentrations than are the larger molecular weight globulins, and fibrinogen which is of extremely large molecular size does not appear in the synovial fluid at all. This relationship is not entirely linear, however, since the large glycoprotein orosomucoid is present in higher concentration than the smaller glycoproteins, haptoglobulin, prothrombin and proconvertin. Large molecular weight substances leave the joint by the lymphatic system and small molecular weight substances are removed from the joint cavity in the synovial veins which drain superficial to bone to the femoral vein.

Joint Lubrication

The characteristic viscosity of synovial fluid is dependent upon the hyaluronate–protein polymerized complexes. This is non-Newtonian viscosity, which means that it decreases with increasing shear rate. Synovial fluid also possesses elastic forces. It seems likely that the viscosity of synovial fluid is concerned in joint lubrication, but the mechanism of joint lubrication is not yet clearly understood there being several alternatives. In boundary lubrication simultaneous deformation of the articulating surfaces and synovial fluid occurs. The synovial fluid film reduces friction by diminishing the tendencies of the surfaces of the cartilage to weld together. In hydrodynamic lubrication the motion of the two surfaces generates a fluid pressure in a wedge of lubricant which forms during movement. The pressure generated in the intervening fluid supports the load on the joint and separates the sliding surfaces. In elastohydrodynamic lubrication it is proposed that both synovial fluid and the articular cartilage contribute to the lubricating mechanism and changes in either impair its integrity. In boosted lubrication it is suggested that the small pits in the surfaces of the articulating cartilage trap pools of synovial fluid thus contributing to the lubricating progress. At present it is not clear to what extent each or any of these mechanisms contributes to the normal lubricating process.

Individual Joints

The individual joints of the body show remarkable adaptation to function. For example, in the shoulder joint the articulating surfaces are poorly aligned and the joint relies upon its surrounding muscles and tendons for stability. This arrangement allows the maximum amount of free movement at the joint. On the other hand, in the hip joint the articulating surfaces of the femoral head and of the acetabulum are of the ball and socket kind, and this arrangement itself confers a large amount of stability upon the joint, while sacrificing mobility.

The structure of the intervertebral disc is quite distinct from other joints. It is composed of incomplete rings of fibrous cartilage, with obliquely running collagen fibres the annullus fibrosus, encircling a soft nucleus pulposus which forms a central mucinous tissue, the whole being well adapted to absorb the compression forces acting upon it. The nucleus pulposus is derived from notochodral cells, and in the adult it is rich in the glycosaminoglycans, chondroitin 4- and 6-sulphate keratosulphate and hyaluronic acid. There are no nerves or blood vessels in the disc, and nutrition is presumably derived from vertebral body blood vessels.

The anatomy and relations of a cervical vertebra is shown in Figure 6 in which the apophyseal joints and the neurocentral joints are demonstrated.

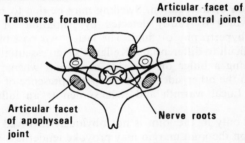

Fig. 6 Anatomy of a cervical vertebra.

In certain joints, such as the knee joint, intra-articular discs and menisci occur. The function of these structures is not entirely understood, but they probably act as shock absorbers. Histologically they are composed of white collagenous fibrous bundles, with fibrocytes, and occasional cartilage cells. In general they are avascular and nerve fibres occur only in their most peripheral parts.

The diarthrodial joint is supplied by blood from the main vessels of the limb by multiple anastamosing vessels. The vasculature of the epiphysis and of the synovial membrane are closely linked and the synovial membrane–cartilage junction is particularly richly supplied.

Development of Joints

Joints develop from mesoderm in the second and third month of intrauterine life. Diarthrodial joints develop as three zones,

9

two dense chondrogenous layers continuous with perichondrium and a middle zone which later liquefies. Synovium, tendons and intra-articular structures develop *in situ*. The final fate and form of joints is determined by functional requirements. Where only limited mobility is necessary the connecting tissue is fibrous (syndesmosis) or cartilage (synchondrosis). Where free movement is required the diarthrodial joint develops.

Clinical Examination of a Diarthrodial Joint

Any history of pain, stiffness and loss of function should be elicited and fully characterized.

Inspection of the joint will disclose gross disease such as subluxation or dislocation. Swelling may be due to bony overgrowth which is readily detected by palpation, or to either synovial hypertrophy or fluid. The latter two possibilities may prove difficult to differentiate. Kellgren's sign essentially consists of observing a bulge on one side of a joint when pressure is applied to the other side, and denotes the presence of a synovial effusion. Local warmth and redness denote an inflammatory process.

If, and only if, the joint is not obviously involved clinically, pressure on the joint margin may provoke tenderness. Similarly, passive movement may reveal restriction in one or all planes denoting clinical involvement, but neither of these procedures should be undertaken lightly in the face of an obviously painful joint. Careful palpation, particularly of the knee joint, may reveal that the seat of disease is not located in the joint, but resides in neighbouring ligaments.

Examination of a joint necessarily includes examination of related muscles which quickly atrophy in the presence of joint disease, of related nerves, and of related tendons which may be dislocated, ruptured, or infiltrated by synovial hypertrophy.

Where indicated, joint assessment may include synovial fluid analysis synovial membrane biopsy, arthroscopy, thermography, radiology and arthrography, and radioisotopic studies and the place of these procedures is discussed with the relevant diseases.

When assessing a patient with arthritis, important points to consider are: Is this a polyarthritis or an oligoarthritis? Is it symmetrical or not? Is it inflammatory or not? Does it effect large or small joints? Are there systemic features? How much does it interfere with the patient's life? How has the patient reacted to his disability? The diagnosis and assessment of the great majority of the arthritides should be accomplished with the minimum of laboratory assistance.

Chapter 3

OSTEOARTHROSIS AND DISC DEGENERATION

Osteoarthrosis is a common disorder of central and peripheral diarthrodial joints characterized by cartilage degeneration, bony eburnation and osteophyte formation.

Disc degeneration is also a common disorder and it frequently coexists with osteoarthrosis, but the pathological changes affect only the fibrocartilage of the intervertebral discs.

Neither is accompanied by constitutional signs or systemic manifestations.

Osteoarthrosis is said to be 'primary' when no aetiological or pathogenetic factors can be discerned, and 'secondary' when there is an identifiable cause. These terms are probably unhelpful since it seems likely that 'primary' osteoarthrosis is a heterogeneous collection of different clinical syndromes, and some of the 'secondary' causes may be merely precipitating or localizing factors. For the sake of uniformity, however, the terms will be retained here.

From epidemiological studies in the United Kingdom it has been estimated that there are approximately five million persons suffering from osteoarthrosis, this disease being the most common of the arthritides. Radiological examination reveals a prevalence of over 80 per cent in the 55 to 64 year age group, and approximately 20 per cent of persons over 50 years have symptoms as a result of the disease. That the disease is by no means confined to the elderly is shown by the fact that in one study 10 per cent of persons aged only 20 years had radiological evidence of osteoarthrosis. Although osteoarthrosis is equally common in males and females, severe disease is more common in females. The symptoms but not the prevalence are more common in cold damp countries than in warm dry areas. Epidemiological studies show an increased incidence of local disease in certain occupations where a single joint is exposed to unusual stress, for example the elbow joint in miners and workers using pneumatic drills, the ankle joint in footballers and the hands in cotton workers.

Clinical Features

Patients complain predominantly of pain and loss of function, and to a lesser extent stiffness.

Pain is usually 'aching' although severe, sudden, excruciating exacerbations may occur at night or after minor trauma. Relationship to weather is common, symptoms being most severe when it is cold and damp, but there is frequently a lack of concordance between symptoms and the severity of radiological changes. Stiffness is usually less severe, of shorter duration, and less clearly related to immobility than in rheumatoid arthritis.

Loss of function in the early stages is related to pain and reflex muscle spasm, but movement may later be prejudiced by joint deformity. However, exuberant osteophyte formation may coexist with remarkable preservation of range of movement.

Absence of any constitutional reaction is a *sine qua non* for the diagnosis of uncomplicated osteoarthrosis. In particular the erythrocyte sedimentation rate should be less than 20 mm/h, the haemoglobin level should be normal and serological tests for rheumatoid factor should be negative. In addition, all differential diagnoses should be considered and rejected, particularly in the cervical and lumbar spine syndromes, since other diseases with a less benign prognosis may coexist with radiologically demonstrable osteoarthrosis and disc disease.

The hands

The joints which are most commonly involved in osteoarthrosis are shown in Figure 7. The pattern of involvement in osteoarthrosis of the hands is shown in Figure 8 where it can be seen that the distribution is quite different from that of rheumatoid arthritis.

Bony swellings of the distal interphalangeal joints, which are called Heberden's nodes, are extremely common. They may affect any or all of the distal interphalangeal joints. It has been suggested that when one or two occur asymmetrically or alone then these are the consequence of a former traumatic incident.

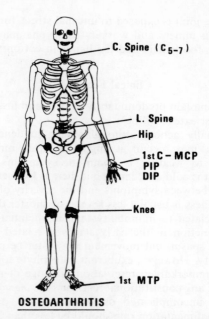

OSTEOARTHRITIS

Fig. 7 Joints most frequently involved in oesteoarthrosis.

Although clinical symptoms as a consequence of Heberden's nodes are remarkable for their rarity, on occasions an acute sudden exacerbation may occur. The affected joint becomes red hot, tender and swollen, and differential diagnosis includes, psoriatic arthritis, sepsis, or even gout.

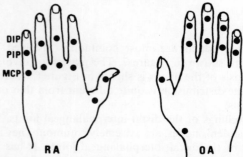

Fig. 8 Distribution of involvement of osteoarthrosis and rheumatoid arthritis in the hand.

14

Symmetrical involvement of the proximal interphalangeal joints occurs in a manner similar to Heberden's nodes, and these swellings are termed Bouchard's nodes. Other joints in the hands and wrists may be affected by osteoarthrosis, including the first carpo-metacarpal in which the disease may be primary or secondary to a malunited Bennet's fracture, and the radiocarpal joint in which involvement is usually secondary to avascular necrosis following a fractured scaphoid. Crepitus and loss of thumb rotation occur with the former.

Two clinical subgroups of primary osteoarthrosis, both involving the hands, have been proposed.

In *primary generalized osteoarthrosis*, which most commonly affects middle-aged females, painful exacerbations in several joints occur successively over several months. All of the above-mentioned joints in the hands may be affected together with the knees and spine. Symmetrical Heberden's nodes formation is usual. Gross osteophytosis is common radiologically but the prognosis appears to be moderately good.

In *erosive osteoarthrosis* a painful monoarthritis of a distal interphalangeal or proximal interphalangeal joint persists for several months. This is then followed by involvement of other joints in the hands, and the knees, the final distribution of involvement being identical to that of ordinary osteoarthrosis. Pathologically a chronic synovitis is found, which may be indistinguishable from rheumatoid arthritis. Although these patients are sero-negative for rheumatoid factor, articular erosions and bone cysts are found on X-ray in addition to osteophytosis and subchondral sclerosis. Before this diagnosis is made all other forms of sero-negative arthritis must be excluded.

Knee joint

Knee joint involvement in osteoarthrosis is similar to involvement of other joints pathologically and radiologically. Prominence of the tibial spines is an early sign and patello-femoral osteoarthrotic changes are frequently seen in younger patients following an ill-defined disease called 'chondromalacia patellae'. As in other joints, but especially in the knee, a chronic synovitis occurs and has been attributed to 'flaking' of diseased cartilage fragments. Knee involvement is particularly common in obesity and in females with maturity onset diabetes. Clinically, quadriceps wasting, a small effusion, crepitus and 'grating' of the patella on the femur occur in early stages and a flexion deformity follows. Tenderness is elicited by pressure over the joint margin or on moving the patella over the femur. In the later stages gross osteophytosis is usual, and a valgus or varus deformity may supervene.

Hip joints

Unlike rheumatoid arthritis, the hip joints are frequently affected in osteoarthrosis and are the source of the greatest pain and disability encountered by patients with this disease. The frequency of involvement is partly due to the many secondary 'causes' or localizing factors operative in this region such as pre-existing arthritis, congenital hip dislocation or dysplasias, Perthe's disease and fractured femur.

Involvement of the hip joint tends to be bilateral and to progress slowly but inexorably, resulting ultimately in flexed adducted and externally rotated hips which pose a truly crippling handicap to the patient. In the early stages pain and limp are the common complaints. Apparent shortening may be detected early but true shortening suggests either femoral head or neck deformity or protrusio acetabuli and is a late finding. Limitation and pain on hip flexion abduction or internal rotation should be sought. A compensatory lumbar lordosis develops and may cause low back pain. Pain from the hip may radiate to, or even be felt entirely in, the knee providing a classical diagnostic pitfall.

Other joints

In the foot, the most commonly affected joint is the first metatarsophalangeal where osteoarthrosis follows hallux rigidus and hallux valgus. The ankle joint is rarely affected unless there has previously been a malunited Pott's fracture. Rarity of involvement is explained on the basis of the strength of the surrounding ligaments.

The acromio-clavicular, sterno-clavicular and costovertebral joints (particularly T1, 11 and 12) are frequently found to be involved histologically, but rarely present a clinical problem during life. Rarely pain due to osteophytosis of a costovertebral joint may be referred around the trunk and may be aggravated by deep breathing requiring differentiation from pleurisy, herpes, angina or cholecystitis. Posterior midline tenderness and pain on antero-posterior pressure may be elicited.

Osteoarthrosis is the most common organic disorder of the temporo-mandibular joint producing pain and 'grating' on jaw movement. Malocclusion is frequently present. Diagnosis is from 'Costen's syndrome', which is a heterogeneous collection of poorly characterized symptom complexes, a common feature of which is facial pain. In the young, symptoms from the temporo-mandibular joint may be produced by developmental abnormalities of the joint which commonly disappear spontaneously. In the elderly, symptoms may be due to loss of support by the molar teeth and may be corrected by dental splints.

In other peripheral joints osteoarthrosis usually occurs only as a consequence of previous injury.

Spinal Osteoarthrosis and Degenerative Disc Disease

Since osteoarthrosis of the spinal diarthrodial joints and degenerative disc disease so frequently coexist, and since both may cause identical clinical features these are considered together. Both are extremely common and show a rising incidence with advancing years. Osteoarthrosis of the spinal diarthrodial joints is present in approximately 20 per cent of patients over the age of 35 years, and over 60 per cent of persons over the age of 35 years have radiological evidence of degenerative disc disease. The discs which are most frequently diseased are the lower cervical and the fourth and fifth lumbar discs, but multiple protrusions are not uncommon. In the cervical spine particularly, there is a lack of concordance between radiological and clinical osteoarthrosis. Radiological evidence of degenerative disc disease is more closely associated with clinical symptoms, particularly in younger patients.

Cervical spine

In the cervical spine, neurological symptoms may be due to *spinal root* compression by apophyseal or neurocentral osteophytosis or by postero-lateral disc protrusion, or they may be due to *spinal cord* compression either by apophyseal osteophytosis or central disc protrusion (Fig. 6). Encroachment by apophyseal or neurocentral osteophytosis or by lateral disc protrusion upon the *vertebral arteries* may also result in neurological symptoms.

Acute cervical disc protrusion is most commonly encountered in young adults and may follow undue strain or a traumatic incident. There is severe neck pain of sudden onset due to nerve root compression and localizing neurological signs develop thereafter. In chronic disc disease or osteophytosis (cervical spondylosis) patients complain of pain which may be worse at night and after neck movement, and may be exacerbated by coughing or sneezing. The onset of neurological signs is usually insidious with weakness of one or both legs, paraesthesia in the arms and, less commonly, root pains, urgency or hesitancy of micturition, Horner's syndrome or nystagmus. The combination of upper motor neurone lesions in the legs and lower motor neurone lesions in the arms with a normal jaw jerk helps to localize the lesion. Anaesthesia and loss of vibration sense and of proprioception in the legs may be present, but sensory signs are often confusing due to secondary involvement of neighbouring roots by fibrosis or vascular impairment, or to the presence of multiple disc lesions. The sensory localizing signs are shown in Figure 9. The biceps tendon reflex is subserved by C56, the radial reflex by C56 and the triceps by C7/T1.

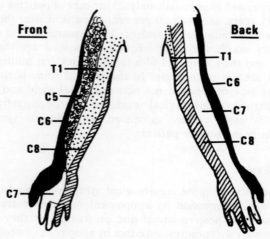

Fig. 9 Sensory innervation of upper limb.

Vertebral artery involvement may present as 'drop attacks' with sudden transient proprioceptive failure often related to neck movements. Rarely a wide variety of neurological signs and symptoms may occur for example vertigo, diplopia, dysarthria, ataxia and cerebellar signs, unilateral paraethesia or hemiplegia.

Differential diagnosis of cervical spondylosis is from referred pain in the shoulder and arm, local lesion of the neck, shoulder or arm (page 161) or neurological diseases. Multiple sclerosis, cervical cord space occupying lesions, motor neurone disease, subacute combined degeneration of the cord and syringomyelia may be mimicked. In any case of doubt, regardless of the presence or absence of radiological changes in the cervical spine, a myelogram should be performed. This should be undertaken in a unit which is equipped to operate immediately since this procedure may actually increase cervical cord compression.

Bedrest, analgesics and immobilization of the neck in flexion in a cervical collar are useful. Manipulation has clamant, but unsubstantiated support and may be dangerous. Heat and massage are widely prescribed and may give symptomatic relief. Vertebral fusion or facetectomy may rarely be indicated when medical management fails, or in the presence of progression of the neurological signs.

Lumbar spine

In the lumbar spine, as opposed to the cervical, spine no major artery is at risk, and the spinal cord ends at L1/2. Postero-lateral disc protrusion producing spinal nerve root compression is more common than is the more serious central protrusion which impinges upon the cauda equina. Acute central disc protrusion producing paraplegia and retention of urine constitutes a medical emergency and demands immediate laminectomy.

Disc protrusion into the vertebral body through the vertebral plate results in the formation of Schmorl's nodes. Lumbar disc protrusion occurs most commonly at L4/5 involving the fifth lumbar nerve root and at L5/S1 where the first sacral nerve root is at risk. The respective sensory localizing signs are shown in Figure 10. Chronic disc protrusion and osteophytosis may produce identical clinical features and are considered together.

Onset of pain is usually gradual, but may be acute following injudicious exercise or trauma. The pain ranges in severity from

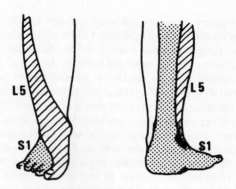

Fig. 10 Sensory innervation of lower limb.

mild diffuse discomfort to an agonizing lancinating pain radiating down the involved dermatome which is made worse by coughing or by movement.

There is loss of the normal lumbar lordosis, muscle spasm, and pain on spinal percussion. Straight leg raising (Lasegue's sign) stretches the sciatic nerve and flexion of the knee with the hip extended stretches the femoral nerve. If pain is produced by the latter manoeuvre the lesion is at L3/4. Sensation is lost on the medial side of leg with L4, on the lateral side of leg with L5, and on the lateral side of the foot with S1, root compression. The knee jerk is lost with L4 lesions and the ankle jerk with S1 lesions. Dorsiflexion of the foot is impaired with L5 and plantar flexion with S1 lesions.

Differential diagnosis is from primary and secondary spinal neoplasms, pelvic neoplasms, trauma, tuberculosis and pyogenic infections, herpes zoster, tabes dorsalis, osteoporosis, osteomalacia, Paget's disease and ankylosing spondylitis. Spondylolisthesis is a bilateral congenital defect in the lamina of the vertebrae in which L5 is thrust forward over the sacrum. Low back pain may occur, but instead of loss there is increase in the normal lumbar lordosis.

Radiologically, narrowing of the disc space, subluxation or apophyseal osteophytosis may be seen. Disc calcification is frequently associated with degenerative disc disease but may also occur in chondrocalcinosis, hyperparathyroidism and haemachromatosis.

Treatment of acute central prolapse is by laminectomy. In chronic disease bedrest on a firm mattress, analgesics and a corset may be sufficient. Physical methods other than rehabilitating exercises are of only symptomatic benefit. Where neurological signs are progressing or medical management fails operation should be considered, but is attended by a high relapse rate. Caution in the avoidance of injudicious strain will assist in the prevention of relapse.

Treatment of Osteoarthrosis

The great majority of patients with osteoarthrosis are only mildly affected. In these circumstances firm reassurance that they have an excellent prognosis will greatly relieve the patient and in many instances this is all that is required.

In those patients who are moderately affected with some pain but little functional disability, reassurance is also appropriate. In addition, however, exercise within the limits of pain will increase muscle power and assist in the preservation of joint stability. Simple common sense measures may yield unexpectedly good returns in individual joints, the best example of this being relief of pain in the hip by the provision of a walking stick held in the opposite hand.

Non-steroidal anti-inflammatory drug therapy may be instituted and the drugs of choice for this are aspirin or indomethacin. Osteoarthrotic patients are commonly elderly and smaller doses of salicylates may provoke salicylism in elderly patients. It is advisable, therefore to warn the patient of the dangers of tinnitus and deafness and to instruct them to reduce the dose immediately these are encountered. Other anti-inflammatory and analgesic compounds such as phenylbutazone, the fenemates and ibuprofen, codeine and paracetamol may be of value either alone or in combination with salicylate therapy. There is no place for gold, chloroquine or systemic corticosteroid or adrenocorticotrophic hormone therapy in osteoarthrosis.

The use of corticosteroid by local injections is widespread in the management of osteoarthrosis. Many other solutions have been similarly employed as local injections, for example local anaesthetics, synthetic lubricants, and even lactic acid. Many elegant studies have been published which demonstrate that any effect obtained by this procedure is comparable to the effect obtainable by local injection of a placebo. Furthermore it has been shown that repeated injections of a corticosteroid into, for example, the knee joint may result in severe joint destruction comparable to that seen in a Charcot's joint. There is therefore no place for the use of repeated local injections of corticosteroid in osteoarthrosis.

There remains a numerically small, but medically very important group of osteoarthrotic patients in whom the arthritis has progressed to the stage of joint destruction. Usually it is the hip or the knee joint which is affected and these patients suffer great pain. The treatment of choice today is surgical. Arthrodesis or osteotomy are the operations which have been advised in the past. However, suitable prostheses are now available for both joints. In the case of the hip joint either a McKee Farrar or a Charnley prosthesis and in the case of the knee joint either an interposition arthroplasty (McIntosh) or a hinge joint (Shier's or a Walldius prosthesis) may be inserted. Sufficient experience has now been gained with hip joint arthroplasties both unilateral and bilateral, to show that the results are commonly very good. Knee joint arthroplasty has proved to be more difficult and has not yet been fully evaluated. These procedures have a very low mortality in experienced hands and the duration of stay in hospital is only of the order of 2 or 3 weeks. Late complications, which are uncommon, include indolent secondary infection, loosening of the prosthesis and sheet-like local calcification.

Pathology and Radiology

Cartilage

It is widely assumed that osteoarthrosis is primarily a disease of the articular cartilage of diarthrodial joints. The initial change in the disease process is not known. Early changes are focal softening of cartilage with loss of metachromasia and of affinity for haematoxylin. Following surface flaking and 'fibrillation' in the superficial layers, deep clefts develop and chondrocytes cluster around the margins of these defects. It is postulated that exposure to synovial fluid lysosomal enzymes, and enzymes from the chondrocytes themselves, thereafter accelerates cartilage destruction which is seen radiologically as loss of joint space. The relevance of destructive enzymes to all forms of arthritis is a burgeoning area of research endeavour at the present time.

One difficulty in describing changes in osteoarthrosis has been to distinguish these changes from senescent effects. Cartilage degenerative changes precede the changes of osteoarthrosis. There are biochemical differences between senescent and osteoarthrotic cartilage. Whereas with advancing years the water content of cartilage is reduced, in osteoarthrosis it is normal or may be slightly increased. The only senescent changes in collagen occurring after the third decade may be increased intermolecular covalent bonding, but in osteoarthrosis there is an increased number of parallel, radially arranged fibres and obvious fibre disruption occurs. In osteoarthrosis there is a disproportionate reduction in chondroitin sulphate with respect to keratosulphate concentration. Thus the changes in osteoarthrotic cartilage may be distinguished from those of senescence.

Synovial fluid

Many abnormalities occur in the synovial fluid in osteoarthrosis. The pH is reduced and the protein concentration, particularly the globulin and fibrinogen fractions, is increased as are also the glycosaminoglycan, sialic acid, lipid and phospholipid concentrations. These changes may be to some extent attributable to an accompanying synovitis. The white cell count may be slightly increased. The volume of synovial fluid is frequently increased and some of the alteration in viscosity which occurs in osteoarthrosis may be attributable to a dilutional effect.

Synovial membrane

The synovial membrane has received less attention than other tissues in osteoarthrosis. The work which has been done, however, shows clearly that there is frequently an accompanying low grade synovitis with chronic inflammatory cell infiltrate, and new blood vessel formation which may produce the elevated intra-articular temperatures and enhanced isotope clearance and accumulation rates reported in osteoarthrosis. Rarely the synovitis may be so severe as to be indistinguishable from rheumatoid arthritis. The difficulty which then arises is to distinguish between osteoarthrosis, and secondary osteoarthrotic changes occurring in a joint which is the seat of a pre-existing seronegative arthritis, and this is frequently impossible. The pathogenesis of synovitis in osteoarthrosis is said to be reaction to debrided cartilage flakes.

Bone

Pari passu with cartilage degeneration and dissolution, the bony radiological hallmarks of osteoarthrosis develop, namely eburnation, remodelling osteophytosis and subarticular cysts. (Fig. 11). The morphological process is of unusually heavy calcium deposition in granulation tissue which is formed in

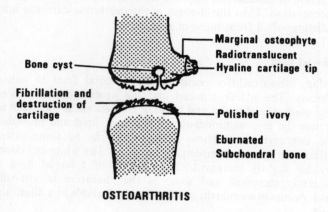

Fig. 11 Pathology of osteoarthrosis.

exposed subchondral bone. This results in the 'polished ivory' or eburnated appearance. Osteophytes develop by enchondral ossification from cartilage–synovial junctions and their leading edge is covered by radio-translucent hyaline cartilage. They may also develop in other areas, for example the 'peaking' of the tibial spines in the knee joint in early osteoarthrosis. High intra-articular pressures are known to develop in joints and are implicated in the development of subchondral bone cysts which have been shown to communicate with the joint cavity. These are in reality pseudo cysts lined by dense fibrous connective tissue and reactive bone. They contain mixed connective tissue elements and fluid.

Aetiology

It is probable that the aetiology of osteoarthrosis is multi-factorial.

Sex and age

That both cartilage degeneration and osteoarthrosis become more common with advancing years is not in doubt. However, there is no evidence that age *per se* is the cause of osteoarthrosis. Thus there are biochemical differences between senescent and osteoarthrotic cartilage. Furthermore not all old people have osteoarthrosis and in those who do there is a wide range of severity of involvement.

In general terms males and females are about equally affected, but severe osteoarthrosis, Heberden's nodes and primary generalized osteoarthrosis, and erosive osteoarthrosis are more common in middle-aged females. Only in the case of Heberden's nodes are the sex differences in any way explicable.

Trauma and obesity

Both excessive use and non-use of joints may predispose to the development of osteoarthrosis. Thus the prevalence of osteoarthrosis is increased in workers, and animals, who use some joints to excess. On the other hand, when a limb is splinted the cartilage atrophies and may later develop oestoarthrosis. Relative immobility, however, exerts a protective effect since Heberden's nodes do not develop in the paralysed limbs of patients who have had poliomyelitis or a cerebrovascular accident.

The preservation of the congruity of the articulating surfaces is likely to be of importance, and this is particularly noticeable in the hip joint. When the congruity of articulating surfaces is lost as a consequence, for example, of pre-existing arthritis, congenital hip dislocation or dysplasias, Perthe's disease or fractures of the femur then osteoarthrosis subsequently develops.

Much has been written about the influence of obesity on osteoarthrosis. The disease affects the obese more commonly than their thinner fellows. However, there is an increased prevalence of Heberden's nodes in obese males, and obesity correlates with the frequency of involvement in the non-weight bearing sternoclavicular joint. In neither instance is the increase in weight likely to exert a direct effect. One strain of mouse which develops both osteoarthrosis and obesity has been studied. The F_1 hybrids of these mice are particularly interesting in that some develop osteoarthrosis without obesity whereas others develop obesity without osteoarthrosis. The relationship between obesity and osteoarthrosis deserves further critical study and is probably complex.

Hormonal and metabolic causes

The occurrence of osteoarthrosis in acromegaly has stimulated the search for a hormonal basis in the aetiology of osteoarthrosis. In acromegaly there is osteophytosis, and in addition the cartilage becomes thickened. However, although many hormones affect cartilage *in vitro*, particularly in unphysiological concentrations, no firm basis for a hormonal factor in the aetiology of osteoarthrosis has been delineated. Currently there is interest in the association between diabetes and both osteoarthrosis of the knee joint and hyperostotic spondylitis, but the relationship remains to be elucidated.

Similarly the occurrence of osteoarthrosis in ochronosis has stimulated an as yet unproductive search for a defect in intermediary metabolism with, possibly, the accumulation of a colourless toxic metabolite in osteoarthrosis. The precise mechanism by which the metabolites in ochronosis cause tissue destruction has yet to be defined. However, over the years a hypertrophic arthritis of the cartilaginous joints of the spine and severe peripheral osteoarthrosis develop. Apart from alkaptonuria, however, no other metabolic defect has been implicated in the aetiology of osteoarthrosis.

Another rare but interesting disease, Kashin-Beck disease, occurs in eastern Siberia and northern China and is probably due to the ingestion of grain contaminated by the fungus *Fusaria sporotrichiella*. An insidious polyarthritis particularly affecting the hands is followed later by a crippling hypertrophic form of osteoarthrosis with marked osteophytosis. The relevance of this disease to osteoarthrosis is not clear.

Genetic causes

Apart from alkaptonuria and a few other rare, genetically determined disorders in which osteoarthrosis develops as a consequence of loss of articular surface congruity, such as congenital hip dislocation Morquio Brailsford disease and the nail–patella syndrome, the only relevant field of genetic study in osteoarthrosis has been that of Heberden's nodes. It has been proposed that transmission of bilateral symmetrical Heberden's nodes may be explained on the basis of an autosomal dominant mechanism with reduced penetrance in the male. However, the statistical analysis of this study has been criticized.

Chapter 4

RHEUMATOID ARTHRITIS—I

Rheumatoid arthritis is a common clinical syndrome characterized by a chronic, inflammatory, symmetrical, peripheral
polyarthritis frequently associated with evidence of systemic
manifestations including subcutaneous nodules, vasculitis,
anaemia, neuropathy and pulmonary and ocular disease.

Like gout the term may well include a heterogeneous collection
of as yet undefined disease entities, and incongruities in reported
prevalence, course, prognosis, response to therapy and influence
of genetic factors lend some support to this suggestion.

Rheumatoid arthritis occurs throughout the world. Seventy
per cent of cases begin between the ages of 25 and 54 and 2 to 4
per cent of the population are affected. Clearly, therefore, the
disease is common and afflicts young adults when they and their
country can least afford it, namely at the peak wage earning years
or, in the case of females, when they are housewives with young
children to look after. There is a female predominance of two or
three to one.

The incidence of objective signs of the disease in the form of
articular erosions is as common in Jamaica as in England showing
that climate has little effect on prevalence. This statement is
supported by the equal incidence of rheumatoid arthritis in the
Blackfeet Indians in Montana and the Pima Indians in Arizona.
The prevalence of clinical symptoms however, is higher in cold
damp, areas demonstrating the effect of climate on clinical
expression.

Clinical Features

Characteristically the onset of rheumatoid arthritis is insidious
and may be preceded by malaise and symptoms of vasomotor

disturbance or by 'intermittent hydrarthrosis' or the carpal tunnel syndrome. A recent upper respiratory infection, or a psychological or traumatic incident may appear to antedate the arthritis, but these precipitating factors may merely be focusing the attention of the patient upon pre-existing disease. The small peripheral joints, the knees and the cervical spine are affected in the early stages of the disease. (Figs. 8, 12). In some patients the onset of the disease may be extremely acute and polyarticular with marked constitutional signs and in a few the onset may be mono-articular and may even remain so for many months.

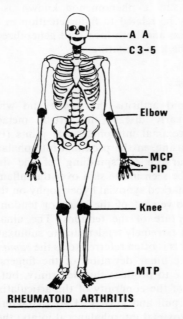

A A
C 3-5
Elbow
MCP
PIP
Knee
MTP

RHEUMATOID ARTHRITIS

Fig. 12 Distribution of involvement in rheumatoid arthritis.

Joint Involvement

Patients complain of pain, stiffness and loss of function in the involved joints. In few diseases do patients suffer such unremitting debilitating pain. There are few pain receptors in cartilage or synovial membrane and pain in inflamed joints probably arises from periarticular tissues, ligaments and tendons.

The chemical mediators of pain and the type of pain receptors in inflamed joints remain to be defined. Pain sensation travels to the spinal cord by fast medullated A fibres and by slow naked C fibres, and thence to the thalamus and cerebral cortex. In rheumatoid arthritis, pain threshold is highly variable from individual to individual and may be influenced by many factors. For example, pain is felt less in warm dry climatic conditions. Patients often complain of stiffness in their joints particularly in the morning, and this is relieved by exercise. In addition, after periods of relative inactivity such as sitting in a chair the joints often become stiff, a phenomenon known as 'gelling'. These symptoms may be related to fluid retention in the periarticular tissues. Stiffness, and both local and generalized weakness may in themselves be incapacitating.

Hands and wrists

In rheumatoid arthritis the hands and wrists are usually involved. In early disease the wrists, metacarpophalangeal (MCP) and proximal interphalangeal joints (PIP) are swollen and tender causing, in the proximal interphalangeal joints, the classical appearance of 'spindling' of the fingers. A dusky cyanosis may be seen in the skin over the inflamed joints. Later there may be marked synovial hypertrophy on the dorsum of the wrist with involvement of the extensor tendon sheaths, which may cause rupture of the tendons. The ulnar head may be prominent and extremely tender, due to subluxation of the ulnar carpal joint. This is often referred to as the *caput ulnae* syndrome.

Characteristic ulnar deviation of the fingers follows. Many factors combine to produce this deformity, but the major ones are alteration of the congruity of the articulating surfaces, displaced tendon pull and gravity. Two characteristic deformities occur in the proximal interphalangeal joints; the button-hole or boutonnière deformity, and the swan-neck deformity (Fig. 13). Involvement of the distal interphalangeal joint (DIP) is rare. A Z-shaped deformity of the thumb is common and synovial hypertrophy may be evident on palpation of the extensor pollicis longus tendon. Wasting of the dorsal inter-osseous muscles is often marked, and rheumatoid arthritis is the most common cause of wasting of the small muscles of the hand.

On the palmar aspect of the wrist synovial hypertrophy may

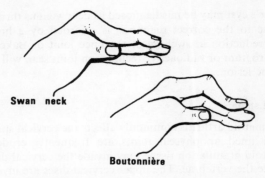

Swan neck

Boutonnière

Fig. 13 Finger deformities in rheumatoid arthritis.

lead to the carpal tunnel syndrome. Less commonly ulnar nerve involvement results in wasting of the hypothenar eminence and loss of sensation on the palmar aspect of the fourth and fifth fingers of the hand. Synovial infiltration of flexor tendon sheaths which may cause a trigger finger. Palmar erythema ('liver palms') is often present in severe disease. Mild vasomotor disturbances in the fingers are common in rheumatoid arthritis. Typical Raynaud's phenomenon may occur, but if severe in the presence of mild arthritis classical Raynaud's phenomenon should raise a suspicion of scleroderma.

Knee joint

Involvement of the knee joint accounts for a great deal of disability. Synovial hypertrophy and effusion are often marked, and the bursae in the popliteal fossa may be swollen and may communicate with the joint cavity. These enlarged bursae are called Baker's cysts. Quadriceps wasting is often marked, even in the early stages of the disease. Flexion contractures may develop and both the cruciate and lateral ligaments may be destroyed, resulting in gross joint instability and valgus or varus deformity.

Rupture of the joint or of a Baker's cyst, as a consequence of the high intra-articular pressures developed during exercise, causes acute pain in the knee radiating into the calf which becomes swollen and tender on pressure. Ankle oedema often develops and Homan's sign is positive. The patient may also have a slight elevation in temperature. Acute rupture of the knee joint or Baker's cyst may be misdiagnosed as deep venous thrombosis. The clue to the correct diagnosis is afforded by a history of sudden reduction in swelling of the knee joint or Baker's cyst. An arthrogram or radioactive technetium joint scan will demonstrate the lesion.

Cervical spine

Rheumatoid arthritis commonly affects the cervical spine. The synovial lined apophyseal joints are frequently eroded, and rheumatoid granulation tissue may invade the cervical discs and penetrate the vertebrae. The upper cervical discs are involved in contradistinction to lower cervical involvement in osteoarthrosis, and gross osteophyte formation is uncommon. The cervical vertebra may be subluxed and this may cause serious neurological sequelae.

The atlanto-axial articulations and their associated ligaments are frequently involved and may become unstable. This is detected by taking lateral X-ray films in both flexion and extension, where separation between the odontoid process and the first cervical vertebra exceeds the normal 2 to 3 mm (Fig. 14). Patients with atlanto-axial disease often complain of pain radiating along the distribution of the first and second cervical nerves. Pain commences in the cervical spine and radiates upwards over the occiput and vertex to the forehead. Symptomatic relief may be afforded by a well fitting cervical collar. To lessen the pain the patient often holds his head flexed or to the side.

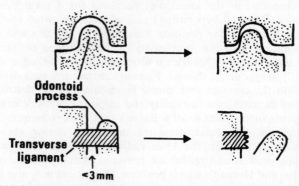

Odontoid process

Transverse ligament

<3 mm

Fig. 14 Atlanto axial subluxation, antero posterior (above) and lateral (below).

Atlanto-axial dislocation may cause vertebrobasilar insufficiency or may produce neurological signs by direct pressure on the cord. However, neurological sequelae from this radiographically terrifying lesion are fortunately less common than might be expected. Since orthopaedic surgery is now common in rheumatoid arthritis patients it is vital that anaesthetists are aware of this potentially fatal lesion, since patients with cervical spine disease are liable to neurological complications with even mild trauma.

Joints of the foot

The ankle joint is less commonly affected than other joints, possibly due to its relative paucity of synovial tissue. Pain in the region of the ankle joint may be due to inflammation of the peroneal tendon sheaths and Achilles tendon bursa or may be caused by involvement of the mid-tarsal joints. Inflammation in the Achilles tendon bursa may be evident radiologically as erosions of the posterior–superior aspect of the calcaneum. When the ankle joint itself is involved there is local tenderness on pressure over the joint margin, and pain is felt particularly on flexion and extension. Pain on inversion and eversion of the foot is caused by involvement of the mid-tarsal joints. Pain in the forefoot is commonly due to downward metatarsal head subluxation (Fig. 15). The patient complains of a feeling of 'walking on pebbles' and the metatarsal heads are readily palpable on the sole of the foot. Surgical treatment of this (Fowler's operation) is gratifying and it is therefore important to diagnose it.

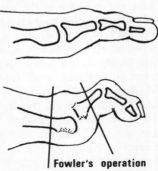

Fowler's operation

Fig. 15 Metatarsal head subluxation (below) with the remedial Fowler's operation. Normal joint (above) shown for comparison.

Shoulder and elbow

The shoulder joint may be the seat of severe pain and limitation of movement in all directions, and involvement of the periarticular tissues is common. There may be tenderness over the bicipital tendon. Rarely the shoulder joint may spontaneously dislocate, or may become completely ankylosed. Flexion contracture of the elbow joint is common and loss of pronation and supination may severely incapacitate the patient. It is important to examine for tenderness over the head of the radius, since excision of the radial head often affords relief of pain and is a simple operation to perform.

Hip joint

The hip joint is less commonly involved than the knee or metatarso-phalangeal joints, but when it occurs it carries with it serious disability. The femoral head may penetrate the acetabulum (*protrusio acetabuli* or 'Otto pelvis') and there may be collapse of the femoral head. This is often referred to as aseptic necrosis and is commoner in corticosteroid treated patients. Patients with severe hip disease not only suffer from severe pain, but also have marked functional disability since they lose both abduction and rotation of the joint.

Other joints

Pain and tenderness are common in the tempero-mandibular joint in rheumatoid arthritis. Sterno-clavicular and acromio-clavicular tenderness may be elicited, but is of little clinical importance since disease in these joints is overshadowed by disease in the larger neighbouring joints. Rarely pain in the throat, hoarseness and stridor may result from involvement of the crico-arytenoid articulations. Involvement of the small synovial lined joints in the ear occurs in rheumatoid arthritis, but does not appear to be a cause of deafness in patients. The sacroiliac joints are, in part, diarthrodial joints and show erosive changes in severe longstanding disease. This is usually unilateral and clinically silent. The apophyseal joints and the costovertebral joints of the spine may be involved, resulting in chest pain which is aggravated by antero-posterior compression.

Constitutional features

Weight loss may be related in part to anorexia, to inadequate diet as a result of iatrogenic dyspepsia, and to increased catabolism of protein. Fever, myalgia, weakness and vasomotor symptoms are common. Depression in the presence of chronic pain is easily understandable and should be specifically sought. Ankle oedema is common even in the absence of local inflammatory joint involvement and may at times be related to disease of the knee causing lymphatic blockage.

Non-articular manifestations

Granulomatous nodules

The commonest non-articular complication of rheumatoid arthritis is the subcutaneous nodule. These nodules are most commonly found over the ulnar near the olecranon process, but may also be found over other bony protuberances or related to tendons, and rarely may occur in pleura, heart, lung tissue, dura mater, or in the sclera. They may arise insidiously or rapidly and commonly remain unchanged for many years. The average size is 1 to 2 cm in diameter, but they may become very large.

Microscopically rheumatoid nodules have a necrotic centre surrounded by a palisading layer of elongated, occasionally multinucleated, connective tissue cells with an outer ring of fibroblasts, lymphocytes and granulation tissue. The necrotic centre is referred to as fibrinoid necrosis. Histochemical, immunological and electron microscopic studies have been conducted on this material which has been shown to consist of a heterogeneous collection of degenerate connective tissue elements, including cellular debris, collagen, fibrin and gammaglobulin. The necrotic centre may liquefy and spontaneously discharge and secondary sepsis may occur. The nodules may heal slowly by fibrosis or may occasionally disappear. When located over bone the rheumatoid nodule may become attached to the periosteum and cause bone erosion. Poor wound healing makes operative removal often difficult.

There is seldom any difficulty in the diagnosis of rheumatoid nodules, although at the elbow the nodules of rheumatic fever, Still's disease, gouty tophi, reticulohistiocytosis, granuloma annulare, and xanthomata may rarely cause confusion. When

35

they occur on the ear they must be differentiated from tophi, epidermal carcinoma and Darwinian tubercles which are cartilagenous malformations.

In early nodules, a consistent histological finding is an arteritis or venulitis at the centre of the lesion. The significance of this finding is at present uncertain, but may be relevant to the pathogenesis of the lesions. Leakage of fibrin or rheumatoid factor—IgG complexes from inflamed vessels may provoke a local tissue response.

Cardiovascular features

Two kinds of arteritis are found in rheumatoid arthritis, namely an inflammatory and a non-inflammatory lesion. Inflammatory vasculitis is common in patients with rheumatoid arthritis. In the majority of patients it is clinically silent, and is only detected by muscle biopsy. Rarely the vasculitis may be indistinguishable from polyarteritis nodosa and may be responsible for such diverse clinical features as peripheral neuropathy, perforation or gangrene of the bowel, dermal infarcts and myocardial or cerebral infarction. It was originally considered that corticosteroid therapy precipitated arteritis since this was seen more commonly in corticosteroid treated patients. However, arteritis not infrequently occurs in the absence of corticosteroid therapy: moreover it is the patient severely afflicted with rheumatoid arthritis who is liable to be treated with corticosteroids and it appears that this is the patient who is also most likely to have arteritis. Venulitis also occurs in rheumatoid arthritis and may lead to venous thrombosis.

The other vascular lesion which patients with rheumatoid arthritis may develop is non-inflammatory intimal hyperplasia of the digital blood vessels, which may lead to digital gangrene. Preceding frank gangrene in the digits, small black dermal infarcts may be seen in the nail bed and nail fold and splinter haemorrhages may occur.

Although pathologists report cardiac abnormalities frequently, heart disease is not usually a prominent clinical problem. Pericarditis, however, may occur in 'malignant rheumatoid', and valvulitis has been reported. Rarely the pulmonary vessels may show changes similar to those seen in the fingers and toes, and may lead to pulmonary hypertension.

Thrombotic thrombocytopenic purpura has been reported in patients with rheumatoid arthritis.

Peripheral neuropathy

Several types of neuropathy may occur in rheumatoid arthritis. In compression or entrapment neuropathy, there is an obvious local cause and the abnormality is confined to one nerve, for example, the carpal tunnel syndrome in which the median nerve is compressed at the wrist. The lateral popliteal nerve and the ulnar nerve may be similarly involved, the former below the knee and the latter at the elbow.

These same nerves may also be involved either alone or in combination in the absence of obvious local causes and this is referred to as mononeuritis multiplex.

In this the more serious type of neuropathy the aetiology is unknown. It may result from arteritis of the vasa nervorum or alternatively may be due to toxic or metabolic factors. It is more common in severe sero-positive disease associated with other complications of rheumatoid arthritis. This neuropathy varies greatly in clinical severity from a mild distal sensory neuropathy detected only by specifically testing the lateral aspects, as opposed to the tips, of the digits with a good prognosis to a severe fulminating sensori-motor neuropathy. In the severe variety, males tend to be more frequently affected than females, the onset is commonly abrupt, and the prognosis for life is poor. The cranial nerves may be affected by rheumatoid neuropathy.

Neuropathy may also occur in patients with rheumatoid arthritis due to crysotherapy or to treatment with chloroquine. Cervical cord compression by subluxation of the atlanto-axial or subaxial joints may produce neurological symptoms.

Amyloidosis

Rheumatoid arthritis is now the commonest cause of amyloidosis in the country, but it is rarely clinically evident during life, and no effective treatment is available. Clinically, therefore, it is of little relevance. Occasionally it may cause hepatic and splenic enlargement or the nephrotic syndrome with renal failure.

Respiratory complications

Pleurisy with effusion is the most common pulmonary complication of rheumatoid arthritis. It occurs most frequently in sero-positive male patients, and is frequently associated with other extra-articular features of the disease. On aspiration the fluid has a high protein content and the glucose content may on occasions be reduced. Rheumatoid and antinuclear factors may be present. The white cell count is elevated and is usually predominantly polymorphonuclear in character. None of these findings is diagnostic and the age and sex of the patient makes it imperative that other causes of effusion are excluded, in particular pulmonary neoplasm and tuberculosis. Effusions usually resolve spontaneously within a month, but occasionally may be persistent. The pleural reaction in rheumatoid arthritis is due to rheumatoid granulation tissue invading the pleural surfaces.

Granulomatous nodules may occur in the lung parenchyma. These are commonly single and present radiologically as 'coin' lesions. As such, differentiation from tuberculoma, carcinoma or lung abscess may be difficult and thoracotomy is advisable in any case of doubt. The histology of these nodules is similar to granulomatous nodules elsewhere in the body. *Caplan's syndrome* consists of unusually large pulmonary nodules in miners with pneumoconiosis who have rheumatoid arthritis or even rheumatoid factor without arthritis. The nodules represent an exaggerated response to the dust disease, and may be related to an altered immune state in these patients.

Diffuse interstitial pulmonary fibrosis rarely complicates rheumatoid arthritis. This complication may be related to deposition of intermediate complexes (page 60) in pulmonary vessels. Patients become dyspnoeic and anoxaemic and develop pulmonary hypertension and cor pulmonale. Respiratory function tests show a restrictive defect with decreased vital capacity, but the ratio of forced expiratory volume to forced vital capacity is normal indicating the absence of airways obstruction. There is a reduction in diffusing capacity. In the later stages severe reduction of arterial oxygen saturation is present. The prognosis for life is poor.

Acute pneumonia is not uncommon in the course of severe rheumatoid arthritis. In many instances an organism can be cultured, but occasionally no organism can be isolated by conventional bacteriological techniques. The prognosis of this complication of rheumatoid arthritis is poor. Some workers have used the term 'rheumatoid pneumonia' for these bacteriologically sterile pneumonias, but the evidence for a specific type of pneumonia in rheumatoid arthritis is lacking.

Patients on long term corticosteroid therapy may develop pulmonary tuberculosis.

Gastro-intestinal, osteoporosis and skin atrophy

Apart from Sjøgren's syndrome, and iatrogenic disease, the gastro-intestinal tract may be involved in the inflammatory vasculitis syndrome leading to perforation, and may also be the seat of amyloidosis. Hepatic 'rheumatoid disease' is clinically insignificant, but lymphocyte and plasma cell infiltrate, brom-sulphthalein retention and raised alkaline phosphatase levels may occur. In some patients focal biliary cirrhosis with positive tests for mitochondrial antibody may be found. Osteoporosis occurs in non-corticosteroid as well as corticosteroid treated rheumatoid arthritis patients. The aetiology has not yet been determined, but it is frequently associated with thin atrophic skin and both may be due to loss of collagen.

Septic arthritis

Septic arthritis may complicate rheumatoid arthritis. The offending organism is usually *Staphylococcus aureus*. Clinical presentation is usually acute with rigors and high swinging temperatures. The septic joint is usually obviously inflamed and aspiration will yield purulent synovial fluid. However, the onset may be insidious, especially in corticosteroid treated patients, and there may be little elevation of temperature and no polymorphonuclear leucocytosis. Diagnosis in these circumstances may be extremely difficult, and can be made only if the physician considers this complication in any ill patient with rheumatoid arthritis or in a patient with a disproportionate degree of inflammation in one jont.

Lymph nodes and spleen

Generalized lymphadenopathy is not common in adult rheumatoid arthritis in contradiction to Still's disease. However local lymph node enlargement is frequently present in regional nodes draining affected joints. The enlarged regional lymph nodes can be demonstrated by lymphangiography and histologically they show simple follicular hyperplasia. Occasionally the follicular hyperplasia is of such a degree as to resemble giant follicular lymphoma or other recitulosis. The position is further complicated by the possibility that tumours of the lymphoid system may be more common in patients with rheumatoid arthritis. It is a wise precaution to biopsy any enlarged lymph nodes above the clavicles or any markedly enlarged node in the axillary, epitrochlear or inguinal regions.

Splenomegaly occurs in roughly 5 per cent of patients with sero-positive rheumatoid arthritis. In some of these patients there is a pancytopenia and the association of pancytopenia splenomegally and rheumatoid arthritis is called Felty's syndrome. The findings in the bone marrow are highly variable ranging from maturation arrest and hypo- or hyperplasia to normal. Assessment of splenic function also has yielded variable results although abnormal localization of radioactive chromium tagged red cells is usual. The haematological features may sometimes remit following splenectomy. It seems likely that Felty's syndrome is not a homogeneous disease entity.

Anaemia

Anaemia is very common in patients with rheumatoid arthritis and is usually of the normochromic normocytic variety. The degree of the anaemia parallels the severity of the disease and improves with suppression of inflammatory activity. The cause of the anaemia is not entirely clear, but it is similar to the anaemia of other chronic diseases such as tuberculosis. The anaemia responds poorly to haematinics. The serum iron is usually low, but the total iron-binding capacity is commonly normal, as is the red cell survival time and the absorption of oral iron. The marrow is normoblastic and contains abundant iron deposits. The synovium also contains large amounts of iron, and it seems likely that there is some degree of malutilization of iron and possibly also a failure of haemoglobin protein synthesis. Interestingly the erythropoetin concentration has been found to be low in rheumatoid arthritis.

Hypochromic microcytic iron deficiency anaemia may also occur in rheumatoid arthritis, especially in females, and chronic loss of blood from the gastro-intestinal tract due to aspirin and other anti-inflammatory drugs may be a contributory factor. This anaemia responds to iron therapy. Rarely macrocytic anaemia occurs in rheumatoid arthritis and may be due to folic acid deficiency. The possibility of drug induced anaemia must always be considered.

Ocular complications

Inflammation of the sclera of the eye occurs in about 1 per cent of patients with rheumatoid arthritis. Usually this presents as a mild episcleritis with congestion of the vessels at the limbus or margin of the cornea (ciliary injection). Scleritis is a more severe manifestation of the same process, and may involve the deeper layers of the sclera and uveal tract. Scleritis is painful and vision may be prejudiced. Rheumatic nodules may occur in the sclera and may lead to perforation of the sclera (*scleromalacia perforans*) and blindness.

Keratoconjunctivitis sicca occurs in roughly 10 to 15 per cent of patients with rheumatoid arthritis. The patients complain of burning and itching in their eyes, which may become inflamed due to secondary infection. Patients may also observe that they do not form tears when they cry. Diagnosis of keratoconjunctivitis sicca is based on an abnormal Schirmer tear test, rose bengal staining of the conjunctivae and slit lamp examination which shows punctate or filamentary keratitis. The dryness of the eyes is due to chronic inflammation of lacrimal and mucus-secreting glands of the eye. In approximately 1 per cent of patients with rheumatoid arthritis, xerostomia is associated with keratoconjunctivitis sicca, and this is due to chronic inflammatory changes in the salivary glands which may become enlarged. Xerostomia may be very annoying, requiring the patient to drink water with her meals in order to swallow. The triad of keratoconjunctivitis sicca, xerostomia and rheumatoid arthritis is termed Sjøgren's syndrome. Keratoconjunctivitis sicca and xerostomia may occur in the absence of rheumatoid arthritis or other connective tissue diseases, and is then referred to as the sicca syndrome.

Laboratory Investigations

Agglutination reactions

Rheumatoid factor (R.F.), (page 61) as tested by either the sheep cell agglutination test or latex particle fixation test, is present in a high proportion of patients with rheumatoid arthritis, but is also found in other arthritides and even in non-arthritic subjects. The test is therefore not diagnostically specific for rheumatoid arthritis. Antinuclear factor is present in approximately 30 per cent of patients with rheumatoid arthritis when tested by the indirect immunofluorescence technique. The pattern of staining is of the homogeneous type, and the antibody is usually to the DNA–histone complex. High serum titres occur especially in severe disease and tend to be associated with a poor prognosis, but do not alone justify the diagnosis of systemic lupus erythematosus. These patients do not develop the renal manifestations of systemic lupus erythematosus. In Felty's syndrome, antinuclear factors may be detected which react specifically with the nuclei of polymorphonuclear leucocytes *in vitro*. There is some evidence that there may be an increase in thyroid autoantibodies in rheumatoid arthritis. There is, however, no evidence of an association with other organ specific autoimmune diseases, such as chronic atrophic gastritis.

As previously mentioned anaemia is frequently encountered with rheumatoid arthritis. Haemoglobin values rarely fall below ten g/100 ml unless there is an associated iron deficiency anaemia. Values less than this merit full investigation. The total white cell count is usually normal in rheumatoid arthritis, but may be elevated during acute exacerbations. Very high white counts should raise the suspicion of infection, in particular of a septic arthritis. Leucopenia is found in Felty's syndrome. Differential white cell counts usually show a mild lymphopenia. The platelet count may be elevated in rheumatoid arthritis, but is usually depressed in Felty's syndrome.

The erythrocyte sedimentation rate may be moderately or even markedly elevated in rheumatoid arthritis, and gives some index of the degree of severity of the disease. However, it is an insensitive index and does not mirror clinical change over short time periods. With corticosteroid therapy the erythrocyte sedimentation rate falls during the first few weeks of treatment, but later rises to its original level. The C-reactive protein is elevated in rheumatoid arthritis and parallels the erythrocyte sedimentation rate. The serum albumin is low and the serum globulin is elevated in rheumatoid arthritis. Electrophoresis shows marked increase in the gammaglobulin fraction, which reflects an increase in all immunoglobulin types. The catabolic rates of albumin Igm and IgG are elevated. The serum complement is normal however providing a contrast with S.L.E. The serum bilirubin is normal, but the serum alkaline phosphatase level is often moderately elevated and the serum transaminase values may be raised. These later abnormalities are associated with focal peribiliary lymphocyte and plasma cell infiltration and mitochondrial autoantibody can sometimes be detected. The serum cholesterol is usually slightly decreased, but synovial fluid levels are often markedly raised.

The serum uric acid level is normal in rheumatoid arthritis, but elevated values are occasionally found in patients receiving aspirin therapy. Other serum biochemical values are normal. Proteinuria and marked renal impairment should suggest the possibility of amyloidosis or analgesic, nephropathy although 'rheumatoid glomerulitis' may occur.

Assessment

The patient should first be asked to give an opinion on the present severity of the disease and upon its general trend in the past. Such is the inadequacy of the assessment methods presently available that this may be the most valuable piece of information obtained. During this interview, the physician can assess the attitude of the patient to the disease and the impact of the disease upon the patient's life.

A clinical assessment is then compiled on the basis of functional status (0 = fully active to 4 = crippled), the number and severity of actively involved joints where severity is usually expressed as a numerical product of pain, tenderness, swelling and stiffness (each graded on a scale where 0 = absent, 1 = mild, 2 = moderate and 3 = severe), the strength of the patient's grip measured by a modified sphygmomanometer cuff, the circumference of the proximal interphalangeal joints measured either by jeweller's rings or by a plastic strain guage and the time that the patient takes to walk a specified distance (usually 50 feet). All of these clinical methods possess both inter- and intra-observer errors which should be quantitated by the physician, and each is better employed as an index of change in disease severity rather than as a static measure. The individual fallibility of each of these assessment methods demands the use of a combination of them and the physician should choose those methods with which he is most familiar.

Laboratory methods of assessment are no more certain than clinical methods. The haemoglobin concentration erythrocyte sedimentation rate, serum iron level, rheumatoid factor titre and plasma protein values will reflect change in disease activity but are slow to respond to acute changes. Radioisotopic methods such as the uptake of intravenously injected radioactive technetium may afford useful clinical information but cannot supplant the more standard clinical assessment methods. Thermography and other indices of temperature changes are currently being investigated. Radiology is of value only in long term assessment and is also subject to inter- and intra-observer error.

Most of these methods are applicable to the assessment of any of the chronic arthritides.

Prognosis

The course and prognosis of rheumatoid arthritis is very variable. In a group of hospital patients followed for 10 years approximately 20 per cent were fit for all activities at the end of this time, 40 per cent were moderately, 30 per cent markedly and 10 per cent entirely crippled. Although, only 10 per cent of patients were crippled functionally, the disease remained active in the majority of cases and the patients were in pain. The prognosis of milder rheumatoid arthritis patients who are not attending hospital may be much better.

Factors which augur a better prognosis include atypical disease, the male sex, absence of erosions or rheumatoid factor, low erythrocyte sedimentation rate, a good initial response to treatment and the absence of visceral manifestations.

Diagnosis

Rheumatic arthritis is diagnosed on a probability scale graded as 'classical', 'definite', 'probable' and 'possible', according to the criteria of the American Rheumatism Association (Appendix).

Essentially, diagnosis rests on the demonstration of the typical symmetrical polyarthritis, seropositivity and joint erosions (Fig. 16). Practically every disease affecting the joints may resemble rheumatoid arthritis.

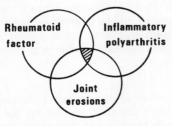

Fig. 16 Venn diagram of the three important criteria for the diagnosis of rheumatoid arthritis. Where all occur in the same patient the diagnosis is 'classical rheumatoid arthritis'.

Treatment

Assessment of any therapy in rheumatoid arthritis is drastically complicated by the spontaneous remissions and exacerbations in disease activity. There is no evidence that joint destruction can be mitigated by currently employed conventional methods of treatment. Although it is incumbent upon the physician to marshal all available resources in the service of his patient the temptation to interfere should be balanced by the paramount consideration of 'primum non nocere'.

General measures

The aim at all times must be to maintain the patient as an independent and useful member of the community either at home or at work. Admission to hospital represents a failure of this primary aim. It must also be remembered that admission of the elderly to hospital may have serious consequences since they may very easily become confused, disorientated and hospital dependent. Moreover, admission to hospital for the employed carries with it the risk of redundancy. On the other hand there is evidence that patients admitted to hospital in the early stages of the disease fare better than those who are not. It has not, however, been established that expert out-patient care would not have had the same effect. Furthermore, it is recognized that patients with disease of acute onset have a better prognosis than those with an insidious onset and the former are more likely to be admitted to hospital early. The decision to hospitalize should not be made lightly and should be tailored to the needs of the individual patients. Hospitalization to tide a patient over a temporary severe exacerbation in disease activity is of unquestioned value.

Rest

It is a general principle that actively inflamed joints should be rested in a position designed to prevent the development of contractures and deformities and this is best done by light plaster cast splinting. It is extremely important that, if hospitalized, the patient should not be totally immobilized since joint contractures may develop. When joints are immobilized in splints the physiotherapist puts them through a full range of movement daily.

It is also important that nurses be aware of the correct use of bed care of a patient with rheumatoid arthritis. When propped up with pillows the neck becomes flexed, and pillows under the knees predispose to the development of flexion contractures. If not prevented, wrist, knee and foot flexion can readily occur. Unfortunately, too many physicians are unaware of the potentially crippling deformities that may result solely from improper bed care. Patients should rest on a firm mattress and have only one pillow at night. The knees should not be flexed, and splints should be applied to prevent wrist and foot drop. An experienced physiotherapist should provide graduated exercises in convalescence to restore muscle tone and joint mobility.

Despite having been shown to have only placebo value, the application of heat in various forms, wax baths, faradism ultrasound and other physical methods is still the common practice in many hospitals in the United Kingdom. Physiotherapy does play an important adjunctive role in the management of patients with rheumatoid arthritis, but the only two measures which are of value are rest and exercise.

Drug therapy

Details of individual drugs are provided in Chapter 16.
Aspirin is the drug of first choice in rheumatoid arthritis on

the basis of efficacy, relative infrequency of serious side-effects and low cost. The main problem of aspirin therapy is dyspepsia, the incidence of which can be reduced by using soluble, enteric coated or glycinated preparations. Recently a polymeric compound of aluminium oxide and aspirin (Aloxiprin) has been shown to produce fewer gastric side effects than conventional aspirin. One of the problems in treating a patient with rheumatoid arthritis is that most conventional preparations of aspirin are formulated as 300 mg tablets which obliges the patients to swallow about 15 tablets a day to achieve an anti-inflammatory effect. This can be circumvented to some extent by prescribing preparations containing larger amounts per tablet such as glycinated aspirin, enteric coated salicylate, and aloxiprin. Soluble preparations of aspirin are in general more palatable than insoluble tablets and for a patient who has to be treated for many years this is an important consideration. When properly

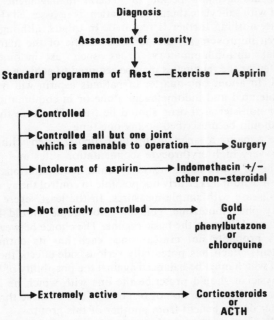

Fig. 17 Assessment and future management of a patient with rheumatoid arthritis.

supervised 70 per cent of patients with rheumatoid arthritis will tolerate adequate doses of aspirin.

It is surprising that it is only within the past few years that it has been appreciated that the dose of aspirin required to be effective in rheumatoid arthritis is 3 or more g per day, and that lower doses do not have any anti-inflammatory effect. In practice aspirin is prescribed to the limit of tolerance. Symptoms of salicylism will be encountered with doses in excess of 4 to 5 g per day, but in the elderly symptoms often appear at lower doses. The toxic dose therefore is close to the therapeutic dose. Measurement of plasma salicylate levels does not provide a sensitive index of overdose. Plasma salicylate concentrations are lower in patients with rheumatoid arthritis than in healthy individuals, and this may be due to lower serum albumin levels in rheumatoid arthritis since salicylates are bound to albumin. Withdrawal of corticosteroid therapy may result in acute salicylate poisoning.

After an *adequate* period of general management supplemented with salicylate therapy the patient is re-assessed (Fig. 17). In some, nothing further is required. In others, although there has been improvement, the addition of one of the many non-steroidal anti-inflammatory drugs such as indomethacin, ibuprofen or the fenamates may be required to achieve complete control. In about one quarter of patients aspirin will not have been tolerated and indomethacin alone or in combination with another non-steroidal drug should be tried. No more than two drugs should be prescribed at any one time.

There remains a small group of patients, often with severe disease, very high erythrocyte sedimentation rates and perhaps with one or more of the extra-articular manifestations of the disease in whom it is clearly not possible to control the symptoms of the disease with simple measures. In the least severe of this category phenylbutazone, gold or chloroquine should be prescribed in addition to the basic regime. The choice between these three is probably not critical since each has its enthusiastic proponents. Each has potentially serious side-effects the likelihood of which must be balanced against the possibility of benefit. The physician should prescribe the one with which he is most familiar. Patients who do not respond to one of these three may thereafter derive benefit from another of this group.

Finally, in the patients who are most severely afflicted by the disease (about 10 per cent) the choice lies between corticosteroids or adrenocorticotrophic hormone. The treatment of rheumatoid arthritis by corticosteroids is empirical and there is no evidence that they affect the ultimate course of the disease. High doses of corticosteroids are no more effective than low doses, but the incidence and severity of side-effects with doses in excess of 7·5 mg prednisolone or equivalent per day are greatly increased. Treatment therefore should begin with 2 or 3 mg prednisolone twice a day increasing to a maximum of 10 mg per day. There is no evidence for superiority of any of the newer synthetic corticosteroids over prednisolone or prednisone. Corticosteroid treatment should be prescribed on a temporary basis at first. Only after it becomes clear that continuous therapy is necessary should this be instituted and even then repeated reassessment is mandatory.

Adrenocorticotrophic hormone, of either biological or synthetic origin may be used in the management of rheumatoid arthritis. It is given by intra-muscular injection. Due to its unselective stimulation of the adrenal there are more mineralocorticoid effects and hypertension, and more hirsutes and other androgenic effects, than with oral corticosteroids. On the other hand corticotrophin does not lead to adrenal suppression, growth is not inhibited, and there is less dyspepsia and gastro-intestinal haemorrhage. There is also less skin atrophy and bruising and probably less osteoporosis, due perhaps to the androgenic effects. A short course of ACTH may tide a patient over a temporary exacerbation in disease activity.

The re-assessment described here should be conducted each time the patient attends for review, the same basic principles being applicable.

Immunosuppressive drugs

Several clinical trials have been reported on the use of penicillamine, azathioprine and cyclophosphamide in rheumatoid arthritis. The results are as yet inconclusive, and at the present time these drugs cannot be recommended for the treatment of rheumatoid arthritis. Conceivably they may prove to be useful in severe progressive 'malignant' rheumatoid disease, although clear superiority over all other forms of therapy will have to be demonstrated since the potential side effects are so serious. More recent results of a controlled long term study provides grounds for guarded optimism.

Intrasynovial therapy

Intra-articular injections of corticosteroids, radioactive gold and thiotepa (triethylenephosphomide) have been used in the treatment of rheumatoid joints. Temporary benefit can be obtained and the risk of infection is small with proper aseptic technique. Intra-articular injections of crystalline preparations of corticosteroids may be complicated shortly after injection by acute joint inflammation due to a crystal synovitis. Repeated injections of corticosteroids, particularly in weight bearing joints, may result in a severe destructive arthropathy resembling a Charcot's arthropathy. Radioactive gold may be useful in the treatment of persistent joint effusions.

Pregnancy

In general, patients with rheumatoid arthritis undergo a remission with pregnancy. In pregnancy it is prudent to use as few drugs as possible and to avoid the use of the newly introduced compounds. Although salicylates have been shown to be terato-genic in certain animals, there is no evidence of such an effect in man, and aspirin remains the drug of choice. Corticosteroids should be continued in low dose throughout the pregnancy; these patients will require corticosteroid cover during labour.

Surgery (Fig. 18)

The most significant advance in the management of patients with rheumatoid arthritis in recent years lies in the judicious intervention of the orthopaedic surgeon. It must be emphasized, however, that scrupulous care is required in selecting patients who will benefit. Of particular importance is the fact that operative intervention must only be recommended to improve function or relieve pain and not for cosmetic reasons. Remarkably good function may be maintained in the presence of apparently crippling deformities, and these patients do not require an operation.

Assessment for surgical intervention is conducted in parallel

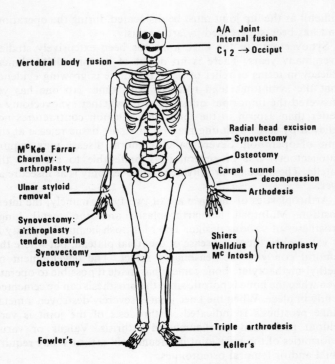

A/A Joint
Internal fusion
$C_{12} \rightarrow$ Occiput

Vertebral body fusion

Radial head excision
Synovectomy

M^CKee Farrar
Charnley:
arthroplasty

Osteotomy

Carpal tunnel
decompression

Ulnar styloid
removal

Arthodesis

Synovectomy:
arthroplasty
tendon clearing

Shiers
Walldius   } Arthroplasty
M^C Intosh

Synovectomy
Osteotomy

Triple arthrodesis

Fowler's

Keller's

Fig. 18 Surgery in rheumatoid arthritis.

with the drug assessment (Fig. 17). The ideal situation is when the patient is generally well controlled, but in one or a few joints there is persistent deterioration despite otherwise adequate anti-inflammatory treatment.

In the hip, where surgery is indicated the most successful procedure is hip arthroplasty, either with the McKee Farrar or Charnley low friction, hip joint prosthesis. It is possible to replace both hips and to restore function virtually to normal. The patient can be discharged from hospital a month after admission. Follow up observations on these arthroplasties over 5 years have revealed no excessive prosthesis wear. The most important complications include infection, dislocation and loosening of the prosthesis, and extensive sheet-like calcification around the joint. Synovectomy of the hip joint is technically difficult as the hip joint must be dislocated during the operation, and has been superceded by arthroplasty.

Synovectomy of the knee joint has been extensively studied over many years. There is no doubt of its immediate clinical efficacy in terms of relief of pain, but there is growing evidence that the symptoms tend to recur with time. No one has yet answered the important question as to whether synovectomy is better than aspirin in the long term. Flexion contractures not relieved by serial splinting may require soft tissue release at the time of operation. Severe patello-femoral disease may require patellectomy, but in general it is preferable to preserve the patella. The place of 'prophylactic' synovectomy is as insecure as ever.

Arthroplasties of the knee are of two types, namely, the interposition McIntosh hemiarthroplasty and the metal hinge prostheses of various design. The McIntosh hemiarthroplasty is of value when there is disease of the tibial plateau, but where the femoral condyles are reasonably intact. The development of methyl-methacrylate bone cement has made it possible to operate even when the bone is porotic since the prosthesis can be cemented firmly in place. When the knee joint is severely destroyed a metal hinge prosthesis is indicated. Arthrodesis of the joint is very seldom performed in rheumatoid arthritis. Valgus or varus deformities of the knee joint in rheumatoid arthritis may require tibial and/or femoral osteotomies.

Painful forefeet due to metatarso phalangeal disease can be readily relieved by excision of the metatarsal heads and the bases of the proximal phalanges (Fowler's operation Fig. 15). Hallux valgus and claw toes are also amenable to surgical correction. Subtalar arthritis can be relieved by a triple arthrodesis.

Synovectomy of the ankle joint is seldom attempted, and arthrodesis of the ankle joint is not a particularly satisfactory procedure. Pain around the ankle joint is usually associated with synovitis of peroneal tendon sheaths, which may be amenable to debridement.

Severe disease of the wrist is best treated by an arthrodesis. The *caput ulnae* syndrome associated with upward dislocation of the ulnar styloid is best relieved by excision of the ulnar styloid. Synovectomy of the wrist is a technically difficult procedure and gives relatively poor results. Synovial hypertrophy of dorsal tendon sheaths or of the extensor pollicis longus tendon requires removal and may be prophylactic in preventing tendon rupture. Swelling of the flexor tendon sheaths may require synovectomy and division of the carpal ligament for the relief of median or ulnar nerve compression. Other operations on the tendons which may be required include tendon repair and transposition for the correction of deformities, and tendon clearing operations for the relief of trigger finger. Z-shape deformity of the thumb is best treated by arthrodesis of the metacarpophalangeal joint in a functional position.

Synovectomy of the metacarpophalangeal and proximal interphalangeal joints has not yet been fully evaluated, but does give impressive early post-operative results. Replacement of these joints by flexible silicone-rubber implants likewise remains to be evaluated. An alternative procedure is the more sophisticated dermal arthroplasty which involves tendon transposition in addition to metacarpal head excision.

Swan-neck deformity may be corrected in the early stages by dividing the lateral bands of the extensor expansion of the proximal interphalangeal joint, but more advanced deformities require an arthroplasty. Advanced boutonniere deformities are more difficult to correct, and usually arthrodesis of the proximal interphalangeal joint in the semi-flexed position is undertaken.

Operative intervention in the shoulder joint is unsatisfactory at present. Synovectomy is liable to be followed by shoulder joint dislocation, and no successful arthroplasty has yet been developed. The simple operation of excision of the head of the radius with or without simultaneous excision of the distal end of the ulna provides gratifying results for the painful elbow. Synovectomy of the elbow joint may be performed, but arthroplasty is still in the experimental stage.

Disease of the cervical spine poses a difficult problem for the surgeon. The natural history of cervical spine rheumatoid involvement is not known, and consequently the indications for surgery are uncertain. However, when severe atlanto-axial subluxation is present and is associated with neurological complications fusion of the first and second cervical spines to the occiput is indicated. Subluxation lower down may be stabilized by an anterior cervical fusion. Fortunately most patients with cervical spine involvement require only a cervical collar.

Finally, it must be emphasized again that many patients present with remarkable deformities who yet manage to maintain adequate function and are pain-free. Such patients do not require surgery.

Chapter 5

RHEUMATOID ARTHRITIS—II

Articular Pathology and Radiology

It should be clearly recognized that the morphological appearances of rheumatoid arthritis are not specific. Pathology therefore affords no certain diagnosis.

The pathological features of rheumatoid arthritis are those of any chronic non-specific inflammatory reaction. The changes are seen first in the synovial membrane.

The earliest recognizable changes are in the small blood vessels. Venular dilatation is followed by stasis, increased permeability and exudation of fluid and cells. In established disease the cellular exudate into the synovial membrane is composed of plasma cells and lymphocytes which may congregate into 'germinal centres'. Polymorphs predominate in synovial fluid. Inclusion bodies in these polymorphonuclear cells have been noted and the cells have been termed 'R:A. cells'. These, however, are not specific for rheumatoid arthritis. Fluid exudation occurs in tissue and also in the joint cavity causing joint effusions. Increased synovial vascular permeability results in an extravasation of large molecular weight substances such as proteins in these effusions. Collections of amorphous material termed 'fibrinoid' accumulate in tissue. This material is seen in many connective tissue disorders and is variously composed of fibrin, immunoglobulin and cellular debris.

The characteristic changes in synovial fluid are a high polymorphonuclear count (2000 to 20,000) and reduced viscosity, the fluid forming a precipitate with acetic acid rather than a clot. In rheological terms the fluid becomes more 'Newtonian' and elastic forces are lost. Glucose concentration may be low, but this is not invariable. The complement level is reduced. Rheumatoid factor is usually present in lower titre than in serum. 'Rice bodies' composed mainly of fibrinogen and cellular debris may form.

Proliferation of the synovial cells results in thickening and fronding of the hyperaemic membrane. Later granulation tissue ('pannus') (Fig. 19) composed of chronic inflammatory cells, fibroblasts and new blood vessels demonstrates virulent invasive pathogenicity probably as a result of the lysosomal enzymes, proteases and polypeptide and amine mediators of the inflammatory response released by these cells (Fig. 24). Lymphocytes, which may be arranged in follicles, and plasma cells predominate

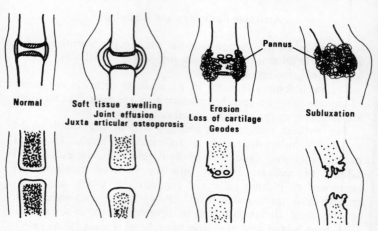

Fig. 19 Pathology (above) and radiology (below) of rheumatoid arthritis.

in the cellular infiltrate. Multi-nucleated giant cells may also be seen. The pannus invades and destroys articular cartilage from the synovial membrane cartilage junction causing erosions on X-ray and spreads medially causing reduction in cartilage which is seen radiologically as loss of 'joint space'.

Possibly due to release of lysosomal or proteolytic enzymes cartilage ground substance loses its metachromatic staining and cartilage lysis follows. Underlying bone is osteoporotic but has been shown by dynamic radioisotopic studies to be the seat of increased calcium turnover. Tendon sheath linings are frequently involved as are pre-existing and newly formed bursae. High pressures are developed inside the joint on movement and this forces synovial fluid into bone forming subarticular bone cysts called geodes.

In the final stages joint destruction, secondary osteoarthrosis, fibrous and even bony ankylosis ensue. Bony ankylosis occurs most frequently in sero-negative patients. Destruction and loss of congruity of the articulating surfaces and tendon displacement or rupture result in subluxations and contribute to the typical deformities which are so characteristic of the disease.

The radiological changes mirror the pathology of the disease (Fig. 19). In the early stages there is soft tissue swelling and juxta-articular osteoporosis. The thin white line of subarticular cortex stands out clearly in relief. Small marginal erosions with irregular edges follow and pannus may extend over the articular surface eroding the white cortical line. At this time loss of joint space mirrors cartilage destruction. Alteration in articular congruity results in subluxations and finally bony ankylosis may follow. Early erosions should be sought in the metatarso-phalangeal joints, wrists and cervical spine as well as in the small joints of the hands.

Aetiology and Pathogenesis

Currently three main possibilities which are by no means mutually exclusive require serious consideration.

Infection

The clinical similarity of some cases of rheumatoid arthritis to an infectious process, and the fact that the rheumatoid factor is produced during the course of many chronic infectious diseases raises the possibility of an infective aetiology in rheumatoid arthritis. Although actively considered in the 1930s this possibility was neglected thereafter for 30 years. Recently, however, interest has been re-awakened by the isolation of diphtheroid organisms and of mycoplasma from joints of patients with rheumatoid arthritis. However, these organisms have also been recovered from the joints of patients with other arthritides, casting doubts on the specificity of these recoveries for rheumatoid arthritis. Mycoplasmas have been shown to be capable of binding rheumatoid factor and they are recognized as animal pathogens which may cause arthritis. However, in considering the significance of the recovery of an organism from a joint, the fact that inflamed synovium acts as a bacterial sieve must be remembered.

The possibility of a viral aetiology is suggested by experiments performed in the United States. Normal and rheumatoid cell lines were established in tissue culture and an attempt was made to infect both with a virus. Whereas the normal cells readily became infected, the rheumatoid cells did not. One possible explanation is that interferon produced as a result of a preceding viral infection was present in the rheumatoid cells. An arthritis, which is transmissible through several generations, has been produced by the injection of cell free filtrates of rheumatoid but not normal syncvial tissue into mice. It is suggested that the responsible agent is a virus. However, these early experiments remain to be validated.

It has been argued that since the incidence of rheumatoid arthritis in the staff of rheumatic diseases is not unduly high then an infective aetiology is unlikely. However, syphilis is an infectious disease with a very low infectivity in later stages and a comparable situation may obtain in rheumatoid arthritis. The incidence of both rheumatoid arthritis and rheumatoid factor is rather higher than expected in spouses, and in relatives of affected patients which could be adduced in support of an infective aetiology.

Although an infective initiating mechanism remains an attractive postulate, no tenable proof of this has yet been offered.

Genetics

Familial aggregation of both rheumatoid arthritis (R.A.) and rheumatoid factor (RF) has been widely reported. However, familial aggregation does not necessarily imply a genetic aetiology: scabies being a disease exhibiting strong familial aggregation in the absence of any major genetic influences. Three pieces of evidence militate against the acceptance of the claims for a major genetic aetiological factor in rheumatoid arthritis: in the family studies reported, the incidence of rheumatoid arthritis in the relatives of patients in some studies is less than the incidence of the disease in relatives of unaffected subjects in others: in one study, where notice was taken of the pitfalls, no familial tendency either for rheumatoid arthritis or for the production of rheumatoid factor was found: no predictable Mendelian pattern of inheritance has emerged despite the fact that the disease is so common.

Further evidence adduced in support of genetic factors in rheumatoid arthritis is contained in pedigree studies. One family is reported in which the disease occurs through seven generations but, since the disease is so common this is explicable on the basis of chance alone.

Twin studies have been used to test the relationship between 'genetic' and 'environmental' factors. The thesis is that if the disease is more common in monozygotic twins than in dizygotic twins, particularly if these monozygotic twins have been living apart, then the probability of genetic influences predominating over environmental ones is increased. Particular dangers lie in ascertainment since there is a bias towards finding and reporting concordant monozygotic twins. In one twin study in rheumatoid arthritis in which most pitfalls could be avoided the maximum possible genetic influence for the disease was calculated at 30 per cent.

In summary, although familial aggregation of rheumatoid arthritis and of rheumatoid factor has been demonstrated, at present there is no evidence for a strong genetic component in the aetiology of rheumatoid arthritis.

Disordered immune response

An immune response may be manifest either as the production of circulating antibody and/or the establishment of a cell mediated or delayed hypersensitivity reaction. Previously, a great deal of attention has been paid to the first of these, but more recently evidence has been accumulating that both may be disturbed in rheumatoid arthritis.

Rheumatoid factor (RF) is an antibody to gamma globulin, and is usually of the IgM (19S) class.

It is generally considered to be an autoantibody, and reacts with the patient's own gammaglobulin. In some patients, however, RF reacts with IgG which possesses different Gm groups from the patients own IgG and in these patients the term *auto*-antibody is inappropriate. RF may react with IgG of human, guinea pig or rabbit origin and occasionally all of these reactions may be detected in the same patient's serum. Generally speaking reaction with rabbit IgG is of more clinical significance than with human IgG producing fewer false positive results. Reaction with human IgG however, is more sensitive and produces fewer false negative results. It may be that rheumatoid factor produced in the early stages of the disease is directed against human IgG whereas later a rheumatoid factor which will cross react with rabbit IgG is manufactured thus explaining the fact that the latex test may be positive prior to the sheep cell agglutination test.

Reaction is facilitated by the heat denaturation of the IgG and it is postulated that this process allows the unmasking of 'buried' determinant groups. The *in vivo* counterpart of this may be denaturation of IgG by some aspect of the disease process itself (Fig. 20).

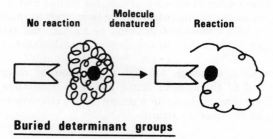

Buried determinant groups

Fig. 20 Reaction of a 'buried determinant' following molecular denaturation by heat or ? by disease.

RF is produced by plasma cells of lymph nodes and in the synovium and may circulate complexed with seven IgG molecules as a 22S complex or dissociated into 7S and 19S fragments (Fig. 21). It has been suggested that intermediate complexes of 11 to 15S formed by an IgG rheumatoid factor and seven IgG molecules, may be implicated in the pathogenesis of vasculitis and of pulmonary fibrosis, and RF itself is known to be capable of becoming attached to the walls of small blood vessels.

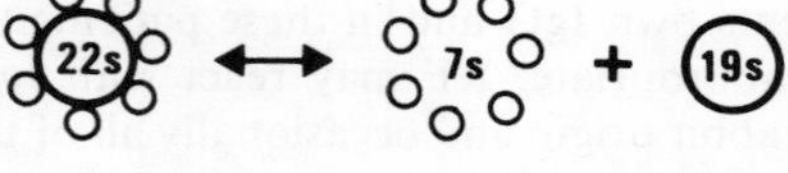

Fig. 21 Physico-chemical characteristics of rheumatoid factor.

Detection of RF in routine laboratories is accomplished by agglutination or by precipitation reactions (Fig. 22). In the agglutination reaction the nature of the carrier particle is not of prime importance. Sheep red cells are used in the more standard sheep cell agglutination test (SSCT), but latex or bentonite particles may be employed. The sensitized IgG may be of human or animal origin and heat aggregated human IgG is used without a carrier particle in the precipitation (F11) test. The result is quantitated by titre.

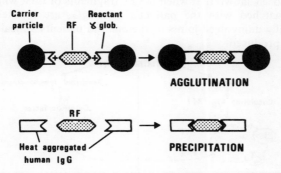

Fig. 22 Routine tests for rheumatoid factor.

The incidence of positive reactions is dependent on the sensitivity of the test system employed and the local laboratory method must be ascertained before clinical significance may be ascribed to the results. With the commonly employed SSCT method the 'cut off' level is taken as 1:32 (Fig. 23) below which

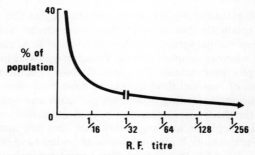

Fig. 23 Rheumatoid factor in the population.

many normal subjects will still have RF activity in their serum. This level is an arbitrary one and the test should be repeated at intervals before categorizing a patient as being sero-negative.

A possible role of RF in the perpetuation of tissue destruction has recently been proposed. It is suggested that complement fixing RF–IgG complexes formed in the synovial fluid may be engulfed by and may then damage polymorphonuclear leucocytes causing a self perpetuating inflammatory response analogous to that seen in crystal arthritis (Fig. 24). In support of this theory it has been shown that when the Fc fragments of IgG, which are Gm matched with the patient's own IgG, are injected into clinically uninvolved joints of rheumatoid patients a local 'flare-up' is produced.

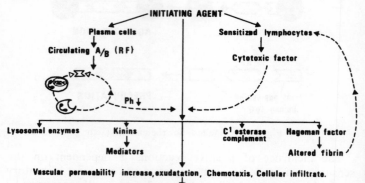

Fig. 24 Diagrammatic summary of the chronic inflammatory response.

The observation remains to be confirmed, but the postulate would explain the low synovial fluid complement levels in the presence of normal serum complement levels in R.A. and also the fact that whereas lymphocytes are found in synovial membrane, polymorphs predominate in synovial fluid. Furthermore the lysosomes of synovial fluid leucocytes have been shown to contain inclusions consisting of immunoglobulins and complement. Against the theory is the fact that oxygen utilization of synovial fluid polymorphs is low suggesting that they are almost non-viable. Furthermore lysosomal inclusion bodies have been found in other arthritides. It is possible that complex deposition occurs not only in synovial fluid but also in the synovium itself and this is currently being studied.

That RF is not primarily concerned in the initiation of R.A. is now almost certain. The infusion of RF does not cause arthritis: not all patients with rheumatoid arthritis have circulating rheumatoid factor; RF may be detected in normal subjects; when IgG with a specific Gm factor is infused into patients known to have a rheumatoid factor directed specifically against IgG with that Gm factor, no decrease in half life of the infused globulin is detectable; red cells coated with IgG react *in vitro*, but not *in vivo* with RF; and finally children with agammaglobulinaemia may develop rheumatoid arthritis with subcutaneous nodules. Although each point on its own may be countered, together they strongly suggest that RF is not the initiator of R.A.

There is, however, good evidence that RF is relevant to the disease process. Thus the disease is more severe and its extra-articular complications are more frequent in the presence of high titre RF. High titre RF activity is recognized as being significant even in the absence of arthritis. In Caplan's syndrome, the presence of RF even in the absence of arthritis is sufficient to produce an excessive reaction to the dust particles.

Apart from RF, antinuclear factor may occur in rheumatoid arthritis which may differ from the IgG antinuclear factor of systemic lupus erythematosus. An antinuclear factor which is specific for granulocytic nuclei is frequently present in Felty's syndrome. However, in uncomplicated rheumatoid arthritis the incidence of other organ specific antibodies is probably not increased.

Cell mediated immunity

Although neglected for many years, abnormalities in the cell mediated immune response are now being described in R.A. The response to dinitrochlorobenzene (DNCB) is reduced in sero-positive rheumatoid arthritis although the tuberculin reaction is normal. There is an increase in the ratio of RNA to DNA in lymphocytes, suggesting increased protein synthesis. Lymphocyte transformation *in vitro* with mitogens such as phytohaemag-glutinin give abnormal results in R.A. It is not known, however, whether these findings are primary or are merely secondary to the disease itself.

Other proposed mechanisms

As in any disease of undetermined aetiology theories abound as to its causation.

Psychosomatic influences have their clamant but uncritical proponents and there is no evidence that endocrine factors are involved in the aetiology of rheumatoid arthritis.

Disturbances of intermediary metabolism have been reported frequently in rheumatoid arthritis. Ascorbic acid metabolism and some aspects of the tyrosine and tryptophan pathways are certainly disturbed but these may be the result rather than the cause of the disease or may even be produced by the drugs used in treating arthritis. The clinical observation that rheumatoid arthritis regresses during pregnancy or jaundice remains to be elucidated, but there is some evidence that this may not be mediated by an effect on cortisol metabolism, as was first considered likely.

An abnormality of the redox system of the lysosomal membrane, which is reversible by vitamin K, has been described recently. The fact that the clinical features of gout resemble those of acute rheumatoid arthritis has been adduced in support of the possibility of metabolic origin for rheumatoid arthritis. These findings do not, however, explain the immunological disturbances.

None of these can currently be upheld as causative factors in rheumatoid arthritis. Currently the theory which is engaging the attention of many workers is that antigen produced by a 'slow virus' is persisting in minute but immunocompetent amounts in synovium and in the genetically susceptible subject this stimulates disease-producing delayed hypersensitivity reactions and disease-marking rheumatoid factor.

Chapter 6

STILL'S DISEASE

Still's disease may be defined as a persistent polyarthritis often associated with lymphadenopathy, fever, skin rash and splenomegally in a child of less than 16 years of age.

The disease is rare, and begins most frequently between 1 and 3 years of age in females. In males there is an even incidence from 2 to 16 years.

Clinical Features

The onset may be entirely articular, the disease presenting as restricted use of a limb rather than pain in the joints, or as a systemic illness with high remittant fever, failure to thrive, growth retardation, lymphadenopathy and a characteristic skin rash (see Table 1). Usually combinations of both presentations are found.

The rash tends to appear in the evening, at the height of the

Table 1 Still's disease (< 16 years)

Polyarthritis—pain, swelling, limitation (two of these) in four or more joints for more than 3 months, or in one joint with biopsy confirmation, other diseases being excluded
Remittent fever
Skin rash
Splenomegally and lymphadenopathy
Uveitis: keratic precipitates, band keratopathy, cataract ⎫
Subcutaneous nodules ⎬10%
Pericarditis ⎭
Complications—infection, amyloidosis

pyrexia, and is a transient, erythematous, macular, 'blotchy' eruption on the trunk and limbs which can be differentiated from that of erythema marginatum by the absence of central pallor and of outward spreading.

The spleen is palpable in one quarter of patients and pericarditis, subcutaneous nodules and uveitis each occur in about 10 per cent of cases.

In the eyes keratic precipitates form as a result of iritis. A separate lesion in the cornea causes band keratopathy. Cataract or glaucoma may supervene (Appendix 2). Expert ophthalmological surveillance is required since the onset of uveitis may only be detected by sequential slit lamp examinations. Generally the uveitis is chronic and insidious with little injection or pain, but in a few male patients more florid changes may occur. It is interesting that some of these patients have subsequently developed classical ankylosing spondylitis in later life.

Subcutaneous nodules are usually situated over the olecranon and histologically may bear a closer similarity to those of rheumatic fever or granuloma annulare than to the nodules of rheumatoid arthritis. Only half of the children with nodules are sero-positive for rheumatoid factor by conventional tests.

The arthropathy most frequently affects the knees, wrists and cervical spine. Distal interphalangeal joint involvement is common, but ulnar deviation is not, providing distinctive differences from adult rheumatoid arthritis. The hip joint is more frequently involved in the child and may constitute a major clinical problem. Whereas the upper cervical spine apophyseal joints are equally frequently affected in adult and childhood disease, fibrous followed by bony ankylosis is rare in the adult and atlanto-axial subluxation is less common in the child.

In some children Still's disease may present initially as a mono-arthritis, and may continue to be localized for many years, generally without any systemic manifestations. In other children tenosynovitis with subsequent tendon contractures may occur in addition to articular disease.

Temporomandibular involvement may lead to micrognathia in later life and this highlights one of the most obvious differences between joint disease in childhood and in the adult, namely the effects of disease on growing bones. Thus both retardation and acceleration of epiphyseal closure may occur, resulting in lengthening or shortening of a limb or digit in adult life.

Laboratory Features

Histological appearances of the synovium may be those of adult rheumatoid arthritis or there may be a mild non-specific synovitis. The greater thickness of cartilage protects the juxta-articular bone from erosive change for longer than in rheumatoid arthritis in adults. Synovial biopsy or even diagnostic synovectomy may be useful in excluding tuberculosis in mono-articular disease, and is mandatory if clinical doubt arises.

Rheumatoid and antinuclear factors are found very much less commonly than in adult disease. Rheumatoid factor tends to occur in older children and augurs a poor prognosis. Patients who are sero-negative tend to remain so.

Radiologically affected joints may show soft tissue swelling and local osteoporosis; periostitis may be observed in early cases. Later erosions, subluxation and even bony ankylosis may be seen. Sacroiliitis is frequently present, but if marked and bilateral may indicate the onset of ankylosing spondylitis. In the cervical spine it is the upper discs and apophyseal joints which are involved.

A normochromic normocytic anaemia, may occur and the platelet count, the polymorphonuclear leucocyte count and the serum globulin level may be elevated.

Differential Diagnosis

Differential diagnosis of articular disease includes trauma, osteomyelitis, tuberculous and septic arthritis, leukaemia, osteochondritis, neoplasm and Morquio's disease. Since joint pain may not be prominent poliomyelitis, scurvy and rickets may be simulated superficially although careful clinical examination will exclude these.

When systemic features are marked at the onset, Still's disease may be confused with drug allergy, sickle cell anaemia, Mediterranean fever and systemic infections. The disease which is most frequently confused with Still's disease is rheumatic fever. The rash and temperature chart, however, are distinctive and in Great Britain rheumatic fever is uncommon before the age of four. Henoch Schonlein purpura may present with fever and poly-arthritis, but again the skin, renal and alimentary signs are distinctive. Dermatomyositis, progressive systemic sclerosis, systemic lupus erythematosus and polyarteritis nodosa may all rarely begin in childhood.

When followed up over many years some children with an initial diagnosis of Still's disease ultimately develop ulcerative colitis, arthritis, psoriatic arthritis or ankylosing spondylitis thus underlining the need to review the diagnosis of these children. In older patients, rheumatoid arthritis may cause confusion. The pattern of involvement, frequency of ankylosis, sero-negativity and stigmata of previous epiphyseal involvement will assist in categorization, but in many instances rheumatoid arthritis and Still's disease are but two facets of the same disease.

Complications

Apart from eye involvement, Still's disease may be complicated by infection and amyloidosis, these being the principal causes of death in the disease. The latter occurs in severe cases characterized by unremittent activity and is usually manifest as proteinuria followed by the nephrotic syndrome.

Prognosis

The prognosis of Still's disease is better than in the adult disease. Sixty-seven of 144 cases had little or no joint residua 10 or more years after the onset of the disease. Early hospital referral is associated with a greatly improved prognosis, but age of onset bears little relationship to ultimate functional capability. In general, females fare less well than males, but on the other hand more male patients later develop ankylosing spondylitis.

Treatment

These children should be referred to a centre which is experienced in the medical, educational and social aspects of the disease. As in adult disease, an assessment of severity and degree of reversibility is followed by the planning of a treatment programme tailored to the needs of the individual child. Adequate local and general rest is balanced against the dangers of immobilization contractures. Serial splinting of reversible deformities must be commenced at the earliest possible moment. A cervical collar may be required. Graded active exercises may be assisted by pool therapy and should be supervised by an experienced physiotherapist. The danger of the effect of chlorine in pool water upon those children with ocular involvement should be remembered.

The principles of anti-inflammatory drug treatment are similar to those of adult arthritis. Aspirin is the initial drug of choice and the dose is adjusted to maintain a serum salicylate level of 25 to 30 mg per cent (80 to 90 mg/kg body weight/day). The usual problems of salicylism in children must be borne in mind.

The indications for other drugs such as gold, phenylbutazone and indomethacin are similar to those applicable in adult disease. Cytotoxic therapy is currently being evaluated. Apart from synovectomy, surgical intervention should be postponed if possible until adult life.

Systemic corticosteroids are especially indicated in the presence of chronic iridocyclitis unresponsive to topical treatment, failure of an *adequate* nonsteroidal treatment regimen or severe systemic disease. One of the most serious side effects of corticosteroids in children is growth retardation which cannot be reversed by growth hormone. Alternate day treatment with prednisolone may reduce this growth retardation as may substitution of adrenocorticotrophic hormone for corticosteroids. Growth will continue on the withdrawal of corticosteroids and if this can be achieved before puberty, the maximum advantage can be taken of the puberty growth phase.

Although peptic ulceration is not common in childhood all of the other adult complications of corticosteroids, or adrenocortico-steroids, or adrenocorticotrophic hormone may be encountered in children, including osteoporosis, posterior subcapsular cataract and suppression of the signs of acute infection.

Scrupulous ophthalmological supervision is mandatory. Symptomatic, mydriatic and local hydrocortisone treatment of uveitis may not be sufficient and the exhibition of systemic corticosteroids may be necessary to prevent blindness.

Intercurrent infection must be treated promptly with appropriate antibiotics. Amyloidosis is probably irreversible, but suppression of disease activity may halt the progression of amyloidosis.

Aetiology

The aetiology of Still's disease is not known. Although erosive inflammatory polyarthritis is more common than expected in female relatives of affected patients and spondylitis and sacrooliitis are more common in the male relatives no clear Mendelian pattern has evolved. No infectious agent has been incriminated and there is less evidence of immunological derangement than in adult disease.

Chapter 7

SYSTEMIC LUPUS ERYTHEMATOSUS (S.L.E.)

Systemic lupus erythematosus (S.L.E.) is an uncommon disease predominantly affecting young females. The aetiology is as yet unknown, although a disturbance of the immune response is probably an important factor, and the diverse clinical features (Table 2) particularly in skin, kidneys, joints, blood, serous membranes, the nervous system and the eye reflect the multisystem involvement which is characteristic of the disease.

The prevalence of S.L.E. is about 4 per 100,000 of the population and over 90 per cent of cases occur in young females, although any age group may be affected. In the elderly, males are more frequently affected, and in this group underlying malignancy may be associated. The disease occurs in all geographical and ethnic groups, but Negroes are more susceptible than Caucasians.

Table 2 Systemic lupus erythematosus

Skin	'Butterfly' rash with erythema, scaling, scarring Drug sensitivity rash
Musculo-skeletal	Polyarthritis; myositis
Renal	'Acute glomerulonephritis'; nephrotic syndrome; hypertension
R.E. system	Lymphadenopathy; splenomegaly
Cardiovascular	Pericarditis; Libman-Sack's valvulitis; Raynaud's phenomenon
Respiratory	Pleural effusion; pleurisy; diffuse interstitial fibrosis
Nervous system	Convulsions; psychosis; peripheral neuritis
Ophthalmological	Cytoid bodies; retinal haemorrhage
Haematological	Normochromic anaemia; Coomb's positive haemolytic anaemia; 'idiopathic' thrombocytopenic purpura

Clinical Manifestations (Table 2)

Skin

An erythematous macular eruption extending across the bridge of the nose to the malar areas on either side in a 'butterfly' distribution is the classical although uncommon manifestation of S.L.E. Photosensitivity is common. The rash is characterized by erythema, scaling and scarring. Minute purpuric elements or telangiectasis may be seen, and in severe cases the eruption may spread to the chest, limbs, palms and finger tips. Alopecia may occur and hypo- and hyper-pigmented areas, bullous lesions or erythema multiforme may be noted. Thrombocytopenic purpura may occur alone or with the erythematous eruption. Dermatological expressions of drug sensitivity are unduly frequent in S.L.E.

The butterfly eruption must be differentiated from acne rosacea in which there are acneiform pustules, rhinophyma and more marked telangiectasis; from seborrhoeic dermatitis in which there is greasy scaling and 'dandruff'; and from the malar flush of mitral stenosis. Histologically there is a capillaritis, hyperkeratotic plugging, acanthosis, and lymphocyte infiltration. Deposits of immunoglobulin and of complement may be demonstrated in both involved and uninvolved skin by immunofluorescent staining.

Musculo-skeletal features

Arthralgia occurs in all cases. In some patients there may be a benign symmetrical peripheral polyarthritis with juxta-articular osteoporosis and soft tissue swelling on X-ray and a non-specific synovitis on synovial membrane biopsy. In a very few patients the arthritis is erosive and deforming, resembling rheumatoid arthritis, but in S.L.E. the non-articular manifestations are more prominent, the antinuclear factor is present in higher titre than the rheumatoid factor, and the serum $\beta 1C$ complement level is lower.

An interstitial polymyositis with vasculitis and some fibrinoid necrosis are found in muscle biopsy in S.L.E. Rarely there may be a marked proximal myopathy.

Renal system

Over 60 per cent of adult patients and an even higher proportion of children with S.L.E. have renal involvement, and this is the most important prognostic factor in the disease. The extent and severity of the renal lesion mirrors the severity of the disease. If renal involvement is absent 2 years after diagnosis then it is unlikely to develop thereafter and the prognosis is greatly improved.

Hypertension, gradually progressive renal failure, a syndrome identical to acute glomerulonephritis, and renal tubular acidosis may occur alone or together. The nephrotic syndrome with low serum cholesterol is said to be particularly characteristic of S.L.E. Renal biopsy is helpful for evaluation of disease severity and may on occasions assist in diagnosis. Acute proliferative changes augur a very poor prognosis. A mild focal or membranous glomerulonephritis may regress and 'light negative' or 'minimal change' findings are attended by a much better outlook. Features characteristic, but not entirely diagnostic of S.L.E. include haematoxylin bodies which are the *in vivo* counterpart of 'L.E. cells', hyaline thrombi, fibrinoid change and a 'wire loop' capillary lesion. Fibro-epithelial crescents are found in severe cases.

The pathogenesis of the renal lesion is largely that of immune complex deposition. The low serum complement is due to deposition of complement and antigen–antibody complexes upon the capillary basement membrane. The complexes are composed of DNA and anti-DNA antibodies and the size and physical characteristics of circulating complexes may be important in determining deposition.

Renal S.L.E. is distinguished from acute post-streptococcal glomerulo-nephritis by the extra renal manifestations, by the presence of antinuclear factor and by the absence of a rise in ASO titre. Post-viral glomerulonephritis and the renal lesions of Sjøgren's syndrome, Goodpasture's syndrome, Henoch Schonlein purpura, polyarteritis nodosa, and scleroderma may also cause confusion.

Haematological features

A mild normochromic normocytic anaemia and elevation of the erythrocyte sedimentation rate are common.

An acquired haemolytic anaemia with a positive Coomb's test may antedate the other manifestations of the disease by many years. This responds well to corticosteroids, but not to splenectomy. The total white cell count is low in S.L.E., but may be elevated in the presence of intercurrent infection. Lymphopenia and polymorpho-nuclear leucopenia with circulating anti-leucocyte agglutinins may co-exist.

A low platelet count with or without antiplatelet agglutinins is common and may be sufficiently low to cause all of the signs and symptoms of idiopathic thrombocytopenic purpura. This also may antedate the other manifestations of S.L.E. Response to splenectomy in this case is usually good. Transfusion reactions are common in S.L.E., and very rarely bleeding may be caused by an acquired circulating anticoagulant.

Reticulo-endothelial system

Lymphadenopathy is common and, if florid, may be clinically and even histologically similar to Hodgkin's disease. Usually only reactive hyperplasia is found histologically. As a part of the reticulo-endothelial system involvement splenomegaly may be detected clinically in about 20 per cent of cases with the classical but not specific 'onion skin' histological picture of concentric periarterial fibrosis. Histological abnormalities found in the thymus include germinal centres and plasma cell infiltration.

Cardiovascular system

Cardiovascular abnormalities are present in over 50 per cent of patients with S.L.E.

A pericarditis with S–T segment elevation and a friction rub is common, but very rarely leads to adhesive pericarditis. Myocarditis with gallop rhythm, extrasystoles, and ECG abnormalities including all grades of heart block may be seen. Cardiomegally is more frequently due to hypertension, however, than to myocarditis. Libman Sacks verrucous endocarditis consists of small warty growths on the mitral and aortic, more commonly than the right heart valves. This occurs in only 10 per cent of cases being the least common of the cardiac complications. The valvular lesions of S.L.E. lead to less disability than do rheumatic valve lesions. Hypertension occurs frequently in S.L.E. and usually, but not always denotes severe renal involvement.

A vasculitis of the arterioles and capillaries may produce digital gangrene, bowel perforation and chronic leg ulceration. Thrombophlebitis also occurs and may be recurrent or migratory raising the suspicion of visceral malignancy. Thrombotic thrombocytopenic purpura may co-exist with S.L.E.

Raynaud's phenomenon is common in S.L.E. True Raynaud's phenomenon denotes regular sequential colour change from blue to white to red and is less common than are non-specific vasomotor symptoms and signs. Digital ulceration and atrophic skin changes may occur.

Respiratory system

Pleurisy, pleural effusions, diffuse interstitial fibrosis and pleuro-pericarditis are the most common pulmonary features of S.L.E., occurring at some stage of the illness in over 50 per cent of cases. Recurrent pneumonitis with scanty physical signs but with radiological evidence of patchy plate-like atalectasis or diffuse basal infiltration may also occur and superadded bacterial infection is common. A wide variety of non-specific functional respiratory abnormalities have been reported.

Abdomen

Anorexia and dyspepsia are common during the acute episodes. Perforation may occur due to arteritis. Dysphagia and motility disorders similar to those found in progressive systemic sclerosis have been described. Hepatomegally may be detected, but overt jaundice should suggest haemolysis. In S.L.E. liver histology shows mainly congestion, and necrosis and cellular infiltration are not prominent.

Nervous system

A wide variety and range of severity of nervous system manifestations may be found in S.L.E. Convulsions of unknown aetiology are not uncommon and may antedate the other manifestations of S.L.E. These may rarely herald the onset of an acute disseminated meningo-encephalitis which may be fatal. Cerebellar and extrapyramidal signs including chorea, cranial nerve lesions and a symmetrical sensorimotor polyneuritis or mononeuritis multiplex may all occur. Although frequently over-looked, psychological abnormalities complicate about one third of cases of S.L.E. and may range from clinically mild symptoms to suicidal depression and psychosis.

Ocular features

Small fluffy white or yellow 'cotton wool' exudates due to localized ganglionic degeneration (cytoid bodies) are particularly characteristic of S.L.E., although they also occur in diabetes, hypertension, subacute bacterial endocarditis, polyarteritis nodosa, progressive systemic sclerosis, dermatomyositis and severe anaemia. Retinal haemorrhages, papilloedema, retinal vein thrombosis, choroiditis and episcleritis may also occur. The Schirmer tear test is normal, but a fluorescin staining keratitis similar to that of Sjøgren's syndrome is common.

In summary, therefore, young female patients with fever, lymphadenopathy, arthritis, a skin rash, serositis, splenomegaly, Raynaud's phenomenon and evidence of renal involvement are likely to have S.L.E.

The conditions which may on occasions enter the differential diagnosis are legion, but important sources of confusion which are treatable are subacute bacterial endocarditis in which there may be fever, cardiac murmurs, splenomegaly, haematuria and pancytopenia, and tuberculosis in which there may be prolonged fever, weight loss, skin rashes, splenomegaly, pancytopenia, and pulmonary lesions. Antinuclear factor is absent from the serum in both of these and absence of antinuclear factor should throw considerable doubt on the diagnosis of S.L.E. Other differential diagnoses have been discussed in terms of specific organ involve-ment.

Features which may antedate the other manifestations of S.L.E. and which should therefore be looked upon with sus-picion, particularly when they occur for the first time in a young female, include convulsions, idiopathic thrombocyto-penic purpura, acquired haemolytic anaemia or even a positive Coomb's test alone, a false positive Wasserman reaction, Raynaud's phenomenon and drug sensitivity.

Diseases which may be associated with S.L.E. include Sjøgren's syndrome, myasthenia gravis 'autoimmune' thyroiditis and in older patients lymphoma or internal malignancy.

Laboratory Findings

The haematological features have previously been described. Serum albumin concentrations may be reduced, there is hypergammaglobulinaemia and the light chains of the immunoglobulin molecule may be found in both serum and urine. Cryoglobulinaemia may be detected, particularly in those patients with Raynaud's phenomenon.

Serum antibodies

The antinuclear antibody responsible for the L.E. cell phenomenon is directed against DNA-histone. The sequence of events resulting in the L.E. cell is illustrated in Figure 25. The antinuclear antibody penetrates the damaged cell membrane of the leucocyte and induces nuclear destruction, shown by swelling

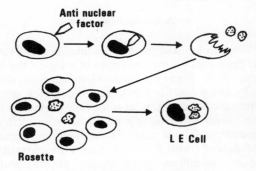

Fig. 25 L.E. cell formation.

and chromatolysis. The leucocyte dies and the altered nucleus is extruded as the L.E. body which is then surrounded by a 'rosette' of polymorphonuclear leucocytes, one of which engulfs the extruded nucleus thus forming the L.E. cell. This must not be confused with the 'tart' cell which is simply a polymorphonuclear leucocyte which has engulfed an undamaged extruded nucleus and which has no clinical significance. The L.E. cell is an *in vitro* phenomenon which has its *in vivo* counterpart in the haemotoxylin body.

L.E. cells are also found in chronic discoid lupus erythematosus, lupoid hepatitis, lymphoma, aplastic anaemia, following the administration of certain drugs and in other connective tissue diseases such as rheumatoid arthritis, progressive systemic sclerosis and dermatomyositis. They are less common and are present in smaller numbers in these other conditions than in S.L.E.

Antinuclear factor consists of a group of immunoglobulins (IgG) which are directed against certain nuclear components. They are detected by the 'sandwich' immunofluorescence technique (Fig. 26). Staining may be observed to be 'homogeneous',

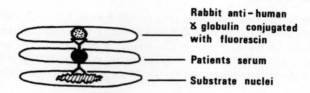

Rabbit anti – human
ᵞ globulin conjugated
with fluorescin

Patients serum

Substrate nuclei

Fig. 26 Indirect fluorescin test.

'speckled', 'nucleolar' and 'shaggy' or 'membranous'. Although doubt has been cast on the specificity of staining the following associations have been reported. Homogeneous staining is produced by an antibody to DNA-histone complex, and is found in all untreated cases of S.L.E. at some time during the course of the disease. 'Speckled' staining is produced by an antibody to an unidentified saline soluble nuclear component and occurs in one quarter of patients with S.L.E. Antibody to deoxyribonucleic acid produces 'membranous' or 'shaggy' staining and usually indicates the presence of S.L.E. with severe renal involvement and hence a poor prognosis. Both free deoxyribonucleic acid, and antibodies to deoxyribonucleic acid may be detected in the serum in S.L.E. Nucleolar staining is produced by antibodies to nucleolar ribonucleic acid-associated protein and is uncommon.

The fact that these anti-nuclear factors cannot penetrate intact cell membranes suggests that they are not the cause of S.L.E., but reduction of serum complement and demonstration of complex deposition upon glomerular basement membrane suggests that they are implicated in the development of the renal lesions.

Other antibodies are found in the sera of patients with S.L.E., including rheumatoid factor, anticytoplasmic antibodies one of which is responsible for the false positive Wasserman reaction, thyroid antibodies, non-specific precipitins and antileucocyte, anti-red cell and anti-platelet antibodies.

Prognosis

Renal failure, neurological involvement and intercurrent infection are the most common causes of death. Although one sixth of patients die within 2 years of diagnosis over 50 per cent of patients will survive for more than 10 years. Complete remissions may occur either spontaneously or with treatment. Thus the prognosis is much better than was formerly believed. It is probable that the reason for this is the early diagnosis of previously undetected mild cases. In general terms males fare better than females and adults better than children. In addition to renal involvement, florid facial eruptions and neurological involvement augur a poor prognosis.

The effect of pregnancy on S.L.E. is variable and if there is no marked renal involvement or hypertension pregnancy is not contra-indicated. Although many of the serum antibodies cross the placenta only anti-leucocyte, anti-platelet and anti-erythro-cyte antibodies produce any measurable effect in the child and even these effects are self-limiting.

Treatment

Patients should avoid strong sunlight since this may provoke exacerbations. It is interesting that ultraviolet light has been shown to be capable of disrupting skin deoxyribonucleic acid and the lysosomal membranes of skin cells. This may explain these exacerbations. In view of the frequency of drug sensitivity, all but the most clearly indicated drugs should be avoided and patients should be warned to take no drugs without a doctor's advice. Simple non-steroidal anti-inflammatory agents are usually sufficient to control the arthritis. Oral administration of antimalarial drugs in low doses (Chloroquine 250 to 300 mg per day) may benefit the skin manifestations, but requires careful ophthalmological supervision and is valueless in the presence of severe progressive disease. High doses of corticosteroids (40 to 60 mg of prednisolone orally daily) are required for haemolytic anaemia, central nervous system involvement and renal involve-ment. Splenectomy may be required for thrombocytopenia.

Intercurrent infection must be treated vigorously with the appropriate antibiotic. Antimetabolites have been employed in severe disease, but have not yet been evaluated. The current consensus of opinion is that the combination of azathioprine and corticosteroids is the treatment of choice for severe renal involvement.

Aetiology

Although great strides have been made in this field, particularly in recent years, neither the aetiology nor the pathogenesis of the disease has yet been determined.

Familial aggregation of S.L.E. and of antinuclear factor occurs but it is not yet clear whether this is due to genetic or to environmental factors.

There seems to be an abnormality of the immune response. Thus, these patients have a remarkable capacity to form antibodies against their own cellular constituents. In particular the renal lesion is produced by the deposition of DNA–anti-DNA complexes and complement on the glomerular basement membrane. The circulating antibodies alone, however, do not damage healthy cells. and do not produce the disease when infused into healthy volunteers, or into a foetus transplacentally. Furthermore, S.L.E. has been reported in patients with agammaglobulinaemia. It seems unlikely therefore that the circulating antibodies are the initiators of the disease.

A defect in the acquisition of immunological tolerance has been demonstrated in a laboratory animal model of the disease and it has been suggested that patients with S.L.E. may have a similar defect with the subsequent production of antibodies against 'self' antigens.

The proposed animal model of S.L.E. is a disease which occurs in New Zealand black mice. Although this disease appears to be transmitted genetically, virus-like particles have been detected and have also been described in human S.L.E. and the possibility of an initiating infective factor in these diseases is currently under investigation.

It seems likely that the aetiology of S.L.E. is complex and multifactorial. Thus for example, either infection or drug ingestion may initiate an alteration in DNA which could then become sufficiently antigenic to induce the formation of antibodies to DNA in an immunologically susceptible subject. Subsequently complexes of the correct biochemical and physical characteristics may form, fix complement and become deposited producing the pathological changes.

Drug Induced Lupus

A syndrome which bears many points of resemblance to S.L.E. occurs in some patients following the ingestion of certain drugs, particularly hydrallazine, procaineamide and anticonvulsant drugs. Hydrallazine induced 'lupus' has been most carefully studied and interestingly this occurs particularly in patients who are 'slow acetylators' of the drug. Although pulmonary manifestations are more prominent and there is a lesser frequency of leucopenia and renal involvement all of the clinical manifestations of S.L.E. have been reported, including the occurrence of antinuclear factor and L.E. cells. The differences may in fact merely represent the age difference in the two groups, the drug induced disease occurring at a later age group. However, the clinically severe form of renal disease does not occur in drug induced lupus. There is some evidence to suggest that those who develop drug induced lupus were already predisposed to the development of the disease. Generally, but not always the symptoms settle on withdrawing the drug.

CHRONIC DISCOID LUPUS ERYTHEMATOSUS

Clinically this affects the face in a 'butterfly' distribution and may spread to the scalp, chest and hands. Erythema and scaling slowly progress outwards leaving a thin central atrophic scar with few talengiectases and alopecia. The buccal mucosa may be involved, and photosensitivity is common. Although only 5 per cent develop florid systemic lupus erythematosus, leucopenia, elevation of the erythrocyte sedimentation rate, antinuclear factor, Raynaud's phenomenon and arthralgia occur in over one third of cases. Some authorities consider discoid L.E. to be 'miniature S.L.E.' and evidence is accumulating to support this contention.

Lupoid hepatitis

The clinical syndrome of 'lupoid hepatitis' consists of recurrent jaundice, arthritis, hypergammaglobulinaemia and the presence of a positive L.E. cell test with homogeneous staining antinuclear factor and positive smooth muscle autoantibody. This occurs most commonly in young females. Biochemical findings include bromsulphthalein dye retention, elevated serum transaminases with normal alkaline phosphatase concentration, hyperbilirubinaemia and hypo-albuminaemia. Histologically there is 'piecemeal' necrosis and plasma cell and lymphocyte infiltration with nodular regeneration and fibrosis in the later stages. Clinical features of portal hypertension and cirrhosis appear in the late stages. Butterfly skin rash, and arthritis are common, but the other features of S.L.E. are not.

On the basis of the rarity of other manifestations, and the different hepatic histology, this disease is separate from S.L.E. but many cases with overlapping features occur. Treatment is with high dose corticosteroids and azathioprine in severely affected progressing cases. Lupoid hepatitis may be associated with Sjøgren's syndrome ulcerative colitis and Hashimoto's disease.

Chapter 8

SJØGREN'S SYNDROME, DERMATOMYOSITIS AND PROGRESSIVE SYSTEMIC SCLEROSIS

SJØGREN'S SYNDROME

This is a chronic low grade inflammation of the lacrimal and salivary glands occurring mainly in middle-aged and elderly females comprising keratoconjunctivitis sicca, xerostomia and, in two thirds of cases, rheumatoid arthritis or another connective tissue disorder. Only two of the triad need be present to make the diagnosis. The presence of the first two features alone is denoted by the term 'sicca syndrome' (see Table 3).

Clinically the patient complains of dry mouth and dry eyes. The symptoms are frequently mild and overshadowed by the accompanying polyarthritis. Stomatitis, parotid or submandibular gland swelling, dysphagia due to masticatory failure and

Table 3 Sjøgren's syndrome

	Triad	Tests
Sicca syndrome	1. Keratoconjunctivitis sicca	1. Schirmer tear test 2. Rose bengal staining 3. Slit lamp—punctate or filamentary keratitis
	2. Xerostomia	1. Salivary flow rate 2. Sialography (sialectasis) 3. Salivary gland scan
	3. Rheumatoid arthritis (or other C.T. disease)	
	± Drug allergy, Raynaud's syndrome, renal tubular acidosis, chronic biliary cirrhosis, purpura (thrombocytopenic or hyperglobulinaemic)	

marked dental caries are more florid manifestations of the disease in the mouth.

Burning, itchiness, grittiness and lack of tears constitute the ocular symptoms, but despite these complaints routine inspection of the eyes frequently reveals no sign of disease or only mild conjunctival injection. Bacterial or fungal secondary infection and corneal ulceration may complicate keratoconjunctivitis sicca.

The clinical features of the accompanying arthropathy are no different from those found in the disease uncomplicated by Sjøgren's syndrome. Involvement of other glands may produce nasal dryness, diminished sweating, pancreatic disease, deafness and pneumonia or atelectasis.

Renal involvement is being recognized increasingly frequently and concentration defects and renal tubular acidosis may be detected. Drug allergy is more common in Sjøgren's syndrome than in the general population, and Raynaud's phenomenon, lymphoid hyperplasia with hepatosplenomegaly, chronic biliary cirrhosis, Hashimoto's disease, chronic atrophic gastritis and thrombocytopenic and hyperglobulinaemic purpura may complicate severe forms of the disease. A predisposition to neoplasms of the reticulo-endothelial system is recognized, and reticulum cell sarcoma, lymphoma and Waldenstrom's macroglobulinaemia may supervene. A fall from elevated to subnormal in the titres of antibodies and concentrations of immunoglobulins may antedate neoplastic change.

Leucopenia and eosinophilia are common although anaemia is rare in Sjøgren's syndrome. The erythrocyte sedimentation rate may be greatly elevated. A polyclonal rise in immunoglobulin levels is common, but can be differentiated from the hyperglobulinaemia of Waldenstrom's macroglobulinaemia and multiple myeloma in which the elevation is always monoclonal.

Sjøgren's syndrome patients have a remarkable ability to produce both organ specific and non-organ specific autoantibodies in abundance. Interestingly, even in patients with the sicca syndrome alone, rheumatoid factor is frequently present. Antinuclear factors with a relative increase in the speckled and nucleolar staining patterns are common and L.E. cells and nonspecific tissue precipitins may be detected. The organ specific autoantibody is the salivary duct autoantibody, but thyroid antibodies and gastric parietal cell antibodies may also be detected. Regrettably the salivary duct antibody is not helpful in diagnosis since it is often absent in the sicca syndrome and frequently present in rheumatoid arthritis patients without Sjøgren's syndrome. It may be more closely related to rheumatoid arthritis than to Sjøgren's syndrome. As in rheumatoid arthritis impaired cell mediated immune responses may be detected in Sjøgren's syndrome.

The definitive test for Sjøgren's syndrome is biopsy of a major salivary gland when diffuse lymphoid infiltration and characteristic epi–myo–epithelial cell islands are seen. This is rarely undertaken in clinical practice, however, and the usual diagnostic tests are sialography which may show punctate, globular or cavitatory sialectasis, measurement of the salivary flow rate both at rest and following lemon juice stimulation and a radioactive technetium salivary gland scan. Normal salivary flow rates do not in themselves exclude the diagnosis of Sjøgren's syndrome, but are none the less helpful in diagnosis.

Ocular involvement is detected by the Schirmer tear test in which the degree of wetting of a filter paper strip subtended from the lower conjunctival fornix is measured in millimetres, at rest and after ammonia stimulation. Rose bengal staining of the conjunctiva delineates superficial abrasions and slip lamp examination reveals a punctate or filamentary keratitis. Punctate or filamentary keratitis occurs only in keratoconjunctivitis sicca and exposure keratitis.

Treatment of the arthritis is along usual lines. Xerostomia is particularly resistant to treatment although a high fluid intake may help. Carboxymethylcellulose eye drops are installed five times per day in an attempt to reduce the complications of keratoconjunctivitis sicca. In resistant cases where residual tear secretion is present, punctal occlusion may help. Topical corticosteroid treatment is beneficial, but increases the liability to local

Table 4 Dermatomyositis

Muscles	Proximal myopathy (polymyositis)	1. Muscle biopsy 2. Muscle enzymes 3. Electromyography
Skin	Heliotropic rash	face (esp. eyelids) over affected muscle

Vasculitis in children; underlying neoplasia in adults.

85

infection. Irradiation of enlarged parotid glands is not advisable since it may increase the risk of malignant change.

The aetiology of this bizarre disease is unknown. Abnormalities of both humoral and cell mediated immune responses are present, but are not yet fully characterized. The initiator of these abnormalities is not known.

DERMATOMYOSITIS

This is a rare disease comprising chronic inflammatory involvement of the skin and of muscles. The term polymyositis is used when skin changes are absent. The joints, gastro-intestinal tract, lungs and heart may all be affected (Table 4).

Clinically the onset is gradual, the disease occurs more commonly in females and there is a peak incidence of the disease in children and again in the fourth to the sixth decade. Vasculitis is prominent in the former, and underlying neoplasia may be present in the cases which occur in later life.

Muscle

The myositis takes the form of a proximal symmetrical weakness and wasting of the limb girdle muscles. The abductors are affected more than the adductors in the lower limb and the extensors more than the flexors in the upper limb. The waddling gait is obvious clinically and on palpation there may be local tenderness or brawny induration of the muscles. The reflexes are reduced and in the later stages the bulbar, but not the ocular muscles may be involved. Contractures develop, particularly in children.

Muscle biopsy histology may be normal, but necrosis, endomysial fibrosis and a chronic inflammatory cell infiltrate may be seen. Regeneration when present helps to distinguish this from the muscular dystrophies. In the child, florid arteritis, with infraction and perivascular cuffing may be seen in bowle, skin and muscles. The serum aldolase and creatine phosphokinases are usually elevated and the transaminase levels may also be raised. Electromyography shows sawtooth spontaneous fibrillation, salvos of repeating action potentials or complex polyphasic patterns. Pseudomyotonic findings may be seen.

Differentiation from muscular dystrophy is aided by the fever,

86

the history of remission and exacerbations and elevated erythrocyte sedimentation rate, but usually muscle biopsy and electromyography are required. In muscular dystrophy there is less
necrosis, no regeneration and no chronic inflammatory cell
infiltrate. The presence of hyperglobulinaemia, rheumatoid factor
or antinuclear factor favours myositis. Skin or visceral disease, if
present, makes the diagnosis of myositis. Differentiation from
myasthenia gravis is on the basis of presence of ocular involvement, more pronounced fatiguability and lack of skin and visceral
disease in the latter. Thyrotoxic, carcinomatous, Cushingoid and
sarcoid myopathy should be excluded.

Skin

The skin manifestations may be almost inapparent or florid.
Classically there is a heliotrope (dark red-purple) discolouration
with oedema and telangiectasis of the butterfly area of the face
and eyelids which may spread to the extensor surface of the
limbs, or may overlie affected muscle. Pigmentation, photosensitivity, sclerodermatous-like change and deep ulcers may all
occur. Ulcers in children may be due to dermal infarction from
the vasculitis and may be very deep and indolent. Subcutaneous
sheet-like calcification may also be seen in children as a late
complication.

Other systems

In about one third of cases there is a mild synovitis of the
knees and small joints of the hands which very rarely may
be erosive mimicking rheumatoid arthritis. Dysphagia and
motility abnormalities similar to those occurring in progressive
systemic sclerosis may be noted and gut perforation due to
vasculitis occurs in children. Rarely there is splenomegaly, but
hepatomegaly does not occur. Pneumonitis, pericarditis,
Raynaud's phenomenon, retinal haemorrhages, and renal
involvement have been recorded.

In some patients the clinical features of the other connective
tissue disorders especially rheumatoid arthritis, Sjögren's
syndrome, progressive systemic sclerosis, polyarteritis and
systemic lupus erythematosus may appear. In adult patients
search for occult neoplasia in the genital tract, lungs, stomach or
blood is wise.

Normochromic normocytic anaemia, eosinophilia, elevation of the erythrocyte sedimentation rate, creatinuria and myoglobinuria may occur in addition to the muscle enzyme elevations and other laboratory findings reported above. Rheumatoid factor and antinuclear factor may be present in low titre and L.E. cells may occur. The muscle enzymes and transaminases are useful indicators of activity and may antedate clinical changes.

About 50 per cent of affected children die within 2 years. In adults the prognosis in those without internal malignancy may be rather more favourable. Treatment is with high dose corticosteroids and is monitored by the muscle enzymes and by the clinical features. In those with malignant disease, removal of the carinoma may be followed by an improved response to corticosteroids.

The aetiology of the disease is unknown. There is no familial aggregation. The associations of some cases with other connective tissue diseases and with neoplasia are interesting, but as yet unexplained. Paramyxoviruses have been recovered from muscle cells of patients with dermatomyositis, but their relationship to the disease has not yet been established. A disorder of cell mediated immunity has recently been proposed.

PROGRESSIVE SYSTEMIC SCLEROSIS (P.S.S.)

This is a rare connective tissue disease which affects the skin, joints, gastro-intestinal tract, lungs and kidneys (Table 5). Females are more commonly affected than males and Negroes more than Caucasians. Onset is usually in the fifth or sixth decade,

Table 5 Progressive systemic sclerosis

Skin	Scleroderma (localized = morphoea)
Musculo-skeletal	Arthritis
	Acroosteolysis
	Soft tissue calcification
	Myositis
Gastro-intestinal	Motility disorders and dilation of oesophagus and colon

± Raynaud's syndrome, renal failure, pulmonary fibrosis

although children may rarely be affected. Raynaud's syndrome or an arthritis very similar to rheumatoid arthritis may precede the disease by many years.

Dermatological features

Localized disease is called morphoea and about 5 per cent of these patients will later develop visceral manifestations (progressive systemic sclerosis). Where the skin lesions are more diffuse the term scleroderma is applied. The face and fingers are particularly affected. In the early stages there is a localized oval, guttate or linear violaceous plaque of atrophic depigmented skin. Oedema and erythema may occur early. It is important to differentiate this from amyloid, chronic oedema, malignancy and a rare self-limiting disease of children which follows an upper respiratory tract infection, sclerederma.

In the later stages of scleroderma the skin slowly becomes tight, producing a 'pinched mouth' facial appearance which may be confused with Parkinson's disease at first glance due to the lack of emotional expression. Skin atrophy, pigmentation, depigmentation, calcification, telangiectasis, reduced sweating, ulceration and gangrene develop insidiously. Hideous deformities of the limbs may develop particularly in the rare instances when the disease begins in childhood.

In scleroderma the skin collagen is neither increased nor abnormal in its constituents although an abnormality of cross linking has been suggested. The protein–glycosaminoglycan moiety, however, is increased in amount. Histologically there is fibrosis, atrophy of secondary appendages and lymphocyte and plasma cell infiltration.

Musculoskeletal system

Acrosteolysis with resorption of the tufts of the terminal phalanges in association with soft tissue calcification is particularly characteristic.

Absorption of the terminal phalanges may occur in other diseases including trauma, Raynaud's syndrome, peripheral vascular disease, peripheral neuropathy, psoriasis, infection, hyperparathyroidism and sarcoid.

Soft tissue calcification may also occur in trauma, chronic

renal failure, hypervitaminosis D, hyper- and hypoparathyroidism, milk alkali syndrome, local infection and dermatomyositis. This must not be confused with myositis ossificans progressiva in which there is sheet like calcification in the musculo-skeletal system associated with congenital abnormalities of the thumb and great toe.

An arthralgia is common, but a symmetrical peripheral polyarthritis may occur with marked morning stiffness. The synovial membrane may be replaced by fibrous tissue. In other cases there may be a synovitis, but there is less erosive change than in rheumatoid arthritis.

The tendons may give rise to leathery 'squeaking' sounds and muscle biopsy shows a focal myositis. In a few cases the myositis may be more generalized and severe and the serum aldolase may be elevated causing confusion with dermatomyositis.

Gastro-intestinal system

In the mouth there may be microstomia, widening of the periodontal membrane and associated Sjøgren's syndrome. Although, all parts of the gastro-intestinal tract may be affected, showing atony and dilatation, the oesophagus is most commonly involved. In 80 per cent of cases there is dysphagia, gastro-oesophageal reflux, or motility disorder. Duodenal and colonic dilatation and diverticulae are common and steatorrhoea, malabsorption and diarrhoea may be troublesome.

Other systems

Raynaud's phenomenon and *pulmonary hypertension* are associated histologically with bland intimal hyperplasia of the small arterioles. Clubbing of the fingers, *pulmonary fibrosis* and 'honeycomb' lung on X-rays are not uncommon, and are associated with a restrictive ventilatory defect, reduced transfer factor or an obstructive defect on pulmonary function studies. In the restrictive defect the vital capacity and total lung capacity are reduced whereas impairment of maximum breathing capacity and forced expiratory volume in one second are most marked in the obstructive defect. Interestingly the incidence of progressive systemic sclerosis is elevated in miners with pneumoconiosis. Alveolar cell carcinoma and cor pulmonale may complicate the pulmonary manifestations of progressive systemic sclerosis.

Renal impairment may be manifest as hypertension, proteinuria and acute or chronic renal failure and histologically focal necrotic infarcts with concentric fibrosis around interlobular arterioles may be seen.

In *the eye,* Sjøgren's syndrome with keratoconjunctivitis sicca may be seen. *Peripheral neuritis* may occur. In *the heart* pericarditis, arrhythmia and electrocardiographic abnormalities may occur. Myocardial and pericardial fibrosis may progress inexorably to congestive cardiac failure which is extremely resistant to treatment.

The disease has been reported in association with dermatomyositis, haemangiomata, Marfan's syndrome and porphyria.

Laboratory Investigations

Normochromic normocytic anaemia is more common than is an acquired haemolytic anaemia with 'cold' agglutinins. Hyperglobulinaemia and elevation of the erythrocyte sedimentation rate are found. Rheumatoid factor is present, usually in low titre, and a 'speckled' antinuclear factor is particularly characteristic although other morphological variants may be found. A young female patient with Raynaud's syndrome who is found to have a 'speckled' antinuclear factor is likely to develop P.S.S. in later years. Cryoglobulinaemia and a false positive Wasserman reaction may be noted. Barium studies particularly barium swallow in the prone position are useful to detect the gastro-intestinal abnormalities.

Prognosis and Treatment

The disease is usually very slowly progressive although remission and exacerbations occur. Sixty per cent of patients are alive 10 years after the diagnosis is made. Poor prognostic signs are marked cardiac or renal disease, severe anaemia, a very high erythrocyte sedimentation rate and high titre rheumatoid factor. Death is usually from renal failure. Treatment is symptomatic. The number of proposed remedies must almost equal the number of physicians who have treated the disease. Currently para-aminobenzoate, and β-aminoproprionitrile are under investigation.

The aetiology is entirely unknown. There is no familial aggregation. The high incidence of the disease in miners has aroused interest in the possibility that silica is involved, but this has not yet been established. Autonomic abnormalities.have been described and elevated urinary kynenurinic acid levels have been reported, but whether these occur as a consequence of the disease rather than a cause is not yet known.

Chapter 9

THE ARTERITIDES

Clinically and pathologically six varieties of inflammatory arteritis are recognized: polyarteritis nodosa, hypersensitivity angiitis, rheumatic fever arteritis, allergic granulomatous arteritis, giant cell temporal arteritis and a miscellaneous group including the arteritis of rheumatoid arthritis, systemic lupus, Henoch Schonlein purpura, serum sickness and dermatomyositis (see Table 6). In the aortic arch syndromes such as Takayasu's disease, in thrombotic thrombocytopenic purpura and in the 'bland intimal hyperplasia' of rheumatoid arthritis and progressive systemic sclerosis, inflammatory cell infiltrate is either inconspicuous or absent and these are considered separately.

Table 6 Arteritis

Inflammatory (Inflammatory cell infiltrate more obvious than necrosis and fibrosis)	1. Polyarteritis nodosa 2. Hypersensitivity angiitis 3. Rheumatic fever arteritis* 4. Allergic granulomatous arteritis 5. Temporal arteritis 6. Miscellaneous—R.A.,* S.L.E.,* dermatomyositis,* Henoch Schonlein purpura, serum sickness
Non-inflammatory (necrosis and fibrosis more obvious than inflammatory cell infiltrate)	1. Endarteritis obliterans of rheumatoid arthritis and progressive systemic sclerosis* 2. Thrombotic thrombocytopenic purpura 3. Aortic arch syndrome

* Described elsewhere.

Polyarteritis Nodosa (Table 7)

This multisystem disease may present with a bewildering variety of clinical manifestations. Particularly suggestive features,

Table 7 Polyarteritis nodosa

Renal	Haematuria, hypertension, 'glomerulonephritis'
Nervous system	Peripheral neuritis, convulsions, subarachnoid haemorrhage
Cardiovascular	Myocardial infarction, arteritis
Gastro-intestinal	Perforation, haemorrhage
Skin	Ecchymosis, 'cropped' nodules
Joints	Polyarthritis

however, are the sudden onset of hypertension, non-streptococcal glomerulonephritis, a sudden symmetrical peripheral poly-neuritis, or a myocardial infarction or cerebrovascular accident in a young person.

Clinically the onset is usually sudden, with fever, weight loss, arthralgia and tachycardia in a young patient. Males are affected more commonly than females in contradistinction to the con-nective tissue disorders. The disease is about one quarter as common as systemic lupus erythematosus.

The kidneys are almost invariably involved and absence of signs of renal disease is a strong point against the diagnosis. Urinalysis is abnormal in over 90 per cent of patients, the most common findings being proteinuria, haematuria or casts. Pathologically there is a focal necrotizing glomerulitis. The arcuate interlobar vessels bear the brunt of the disease with cellular infiltration thrombosis, micro-aneurisms, haemorrhages and infarction. Renal vein thrombosis may occur. Although the blood pressure may be normal in the early stages, hypertension is the rule later on.

Renal failure is the most common cause of death, and is followed in frequency by cardiac failure due to hypertension or myocardial infarction. Pericarditis and cardiac arrhythmias may occur. Bowel infarction, peripheral gangrene and perforation may be fatal. Acute pancreatitis and steatorrhoea are less com-mon gastro-intestinal manifestations. Mononeuritis multiplex or an acute symmetrical peripheral neuritis affecting the lower more than the upper limbs and the motor fibres before the sensory ones may occur. Convulsions, psychoses, hemiplegia and subarachnoid haemorrhage denote involvement of the central nervous system which accounts for approximately 20 per cent of deaths from this disease.

In the joints there may be an acute migratory self-limiting polyarthritis or rarely the arthritis may be erosive and destructive with marked synovial hypertrophy mimicking rheumatoid arthritis. Involvement of skin blood vessels causes ecchymoses arranged in clusters, and subcutaneous nodules which may be pulsatile or may be similar to the skin lesions of erythema nodosum. Involvement of the ophthalmic artery may result in blindness and scleritis and keratitis have been reported. Pulmonary involvement is very much less common than in hypersensitivity angiitis, but pulmonary infiltrates, consolidation and miliary mottling may be seen.

Laboratory findings include a moderate normochromic normocytic anaemia, elevation of the erythrocyte sedimentation rate, polymorphonuclear leucocytosis, cryoglobulinaemia and macroglobulinaemia. Rheumatoid factor may be detectable in the serum. High titre rheumatoid factor, however, suggests that the primary disease is rheumatoid arthritis. The eosinophil count may be raised but is less markedly elevated than in hypersensitivity angiitis or Loeffler's syndrome. Skeletal muscle biopsy is positive in a disappointingly small proportion of cases, but does serve to exclude such rarities as trichinosis. Renal biopsy may be helpful, but carries an appreciable hazard of haemorrhage. Renal angiography may show aneurysms of the renal or intrarenal vessels and should be done first.

The prognosis of polyarteritis nodosa is grave, virtually all severely affected patients dying within 2 years of the diagnosis. Death is usually from renal or cardiac failure, cerebrovascular accident or gut perforation.

The aetiology of polyarteritis nodosa is entirely unknown. Clinical and pathological similarities to serum sickness suggest an allergic basis, and angiitis can be produced by many drugs such as sulphonamides, penicillin, thioracils, phenylhydantoin and arsenic as well as foreign serum itself. However, evidence for hypersensitivity in the aetiology of polyarteritis nodosa is as yet lacking. Some authorities have suggested that all of the lesions of polyarteritis nodosa may be explicable on the basis of hypertensive disease itself, but normotensive cases of polyarteritis nodosa are not uncommon in early disease.

The pathological features of the lesions which occur in medium sized and small arteries, are fibrinoid necrosis, oedema, polymorphonuclear leucocyte and chronic inflammatory cell infiltrate of the vessel wall. Later thrombosis, aneurisms and infarctions are seen. Lesions are discrete and tend to occur at bifurcations.

Hypersensitivity angiitis differs from classical polyarteritis nodosa in being more commonly directly associated with drugs, in affecting smaller vessels and not specifically at bifurcations, in affecting the kidneys and gut less and the lungs more obviously, and in possessing a much more favourable prognosis following the acute episode. Pathologically the lesions show less tendency to heal and are all at the same stage of evolution.

Allergic granulomatosus exhibits more necrosis and granuloma formation pathologically than in polyarteritis or hypersensitivity angiitis. The lungs bear the brunt of the disease with asthma, pneumonitis and eosinophilia. When migratory patchy pulmonary infiltrates are associated with marked eosinophilia in sputum and blood, the eponymous title 'Loeffler's syndrome' is applied. Clinically there is fever, cough and wheeze which respond to corticosteroids. Asthma may be simulated. The syndrome may occur in association with helminth infestation or drug ingestion, particularly penicillin, streptomycin and para-aminosalicylic acid. Renal failure may occur.

In Wegener's granulomatosus the upper and lower respiratory tract are the seat of aggressive necrotic granulomatous lesions. There is usually a generalized necrotizing angiitis and renal involvement is common. This disease is probably related to lethal midline granuloma which affects the mediastinum and face and both are usually fatal. Both diseases occur in the fifth decade, and in both the lesions are locally destructive to adjoining tissues, even bone. Retro-orbital lesions may cause exophthalmos. Generalized involvement with manifestations in joints, heart, nervous system and alimentary system may occur, but death is usually from respiratory or renal failure.

Differential diagnosis is from neoplasm, fungal disease, tuberculosis and Goodpasture's syndrome, which is a fatal disease of lungs and kidneys occurring in young males.

TEMPORAL ARTERITIS

This is a giant cell granulomatous lesion which principally affects the temporal arteries producing local pain and tenderness. It commonly progresses to occlusion of the vessel. Clinically it is important to exclude concomitant involvement of the ophthalmic vessels since this may rapidly lead to blindness. Preceding visual symptoms such as 'flashing lights' in front of the eyes should be specifically sought. The coronary vessels may also be involved. Articular and muscular complaints are much less prominent than in polymyalgia rheumatica, and visceral involvement is less marked than in polyarteritis nodosa. Treatment is with a short course of corticosteroids in high doses, and is monitored by the clinical features and by the erythrocyte sedimentation rate.

AORTIC ARCH SYNDROMES

In Takayasu's syndrome which is a disease of young females the arteries of the aortic arch are affected, producing occlusion of the radial pulse and also of the carotid vessels. There may be claudication in the upper limbs, hypertension, cataract, dizziness, dissecting aneurism and cerebral vascular insufficiency. The vessel walls are the seat of necrosis and fibrosis with less cellular infiltrate than in the other arteritic syndromes, although a few giant cells may be seen.

THROMBOTIC THROMBOCYTOPENIC PURPURA

This is an uncommon disease characterized by pyrexia, haemolytic anaemia, thrombocytopenia and neurological involvement. In the small blood vessels of the heart, pancreas, spleen, liver, kidney and bone there are platelet thrombi, micro-aneurysms and non-inflammatory fibrinoid necrosis of the wall. The lungs and skin vessels are spared and in the diseased vessels there is an absence of inflammatory reaction.

Males and females are equally affected and the course of the disease varies from an acute explosive onset with death within weeks, to a chronic course with remission and exacerbations which nevertheless ultimately leads to death.

Thrombyocytopenia results in petechial haemorrhages, epistaxis, haemoptysis, vaginal bleeding and hemiplegia. Neurological involvement in the disease may lead to convulsions, focal signs or death. Hepatosplenomegaly may occur. The aetiology of the disease is not yet known. The lesion in small blood vessels is thought to result in platelet thrombi and irregularity of the wall may damage red blood cells in transit and account for the bizarre shapes seen on peripheral blood films ('burr cells'). The same mechanism may account for the defibrination syndrome and clotting factor consumption which contribute to the clinical manifestations of the disease. The disease has been reported in association with drug ingestion (penicillin, sulphonamides or iodine) and also with systemic lupus erythematosus and rheumatoid arthritis.

HENOCH SCHONLEIN PURPURA

This uncommon disease of unknown aetiology is essentially a vasculitis which is particularly manifest in skin, intestines, joints and kidneys.

Onset is acute and commonly occurs between 2 and 15 years of age although adults may be affected. Symmetrical small round or oval purple papules, which do not blanch on pressure, develop on the lower legs, feet, buttocks and occasionally the arms. These may coalesce to form echymoses or rarely urticarial lesions. Colicky abdominal pain and fresh bleeding per rectum are common and on occasions an intussusception may occur. A benign self-limiting non-migratory arthritis affects the knees and ankles more commonly than the wrists, elbows or hips. Synovial fluid analysis shows a polymorphonuclear leucocytosis. Renal involvement manifest by haematuria, proteinuria or hypertension occurs in half of the patients and 5 per cent develop an acute glomerulonephritis. Subarachnoid haemorrhage or convulsions are rare.

The erythrocyte sedimentation rate is elevated, the anti-streptolysin 0 titre is normal, as are the coagulation tests, but the Hess test is positive. Histologically the small blood vessels are found to be the seat of an inflammatory cell infiltrate. Thrombosis and haemorrhages are common. The prognosis is good, although a few patients die in renal failure, or with neurological involvement. Symptomatic treatment is indicated and corticosteroids may benefit the severely ill patient. Although 'allergic' factors are mooted in the aetiology of the disease there is no good incriminating evidence for this. A relationship to prior streptococcal infection has not yet been established.

SERUM SICKNESS

From 2 to 16 days after exposure to foreign serum the patient becomes ill with an itchy urticarial rash, lymphadenopathy, fever, polyneuropathy, oliguria and arthralgia. The medium sized joints are involved. Histologically there is a non-specific acute synovitis and a widespread vasculitis. A false positive Paul Bunnell test may be found, the erythrocyte sedimentation rate is elevated and there is a neutrophil polymorphonuclear leucocytosis. Antigen–antibody complex formation with release of chemical mediators of inflammation constitutes the pathogenetic mechanism and treatment is with corticosteroids and antihistamines.

This is differentiated from the immediate hypersensitivity reaction to foreign serum pathogenetically by the participation of IgE in the latter. In immediate reactions there is usually a history of eczema, asthma or other allergy, the time course is much faster and smaller quantities of antigen are required to produce the disease.

Chapter 10

RHEUMATIC FEVER

Rheumatic fever is a connective tissue disease of declining incidence which affects young persons and which is caused by an abnormal reaction of the individual to infection with β-haemolytic steptococcus.

Clinical Features

The disease is characterized by sustained pyrexia, flitting polyarthritis, pancarditis, subcutaneous nodules, chorea and erythema marginatum (Table 8).

Table 8 Rheumatic fever

Fever (sustained)
Polyarthritis (migratory)
Pancarditis
Subcutaneous nodules
Erythema marginatum
Chorea
Evidence of recent streptococcal infection
Elevated erythrocyte sedimentation rate

The onset is acute and follows a β haemolytic streptococcal throat infection by 1 to 2 weeks. Males and females are equally affected and the first episode usually occurs between the ages of 5 and 15. Whereas in children the carditis usually predominates, when adults are affected arthritis frequently overshadows the carditis. The fever is sustained as opposed to the remittent temperature chart of Still's disease.

The arthritis affects large joints such as the knees, wrists, ankles and elbows rather than the small joints of the hands, and is migratory, appearing in one joint and disappearing while it flares up in another. Synovial membrane histology reveals an acute non-specific synovitis with oedema, congestion, polymorphonuclear leucocyte infiltrate, synovial hypertrophy, but with little necrosis or fibrosis. The periarticular tissues may be more prominently involved than the synovium. Synovial fluid protein concentrations are slightly increased and the white cell count is raised. The arthritis is self-limiting and leaves no residual joint damage. An excessively rare syndrome, Jaccoud's arthritis, may follow severe and repeated episodes of rheumatic fever. There is marked ulnar deviation, with flexion of the metacarpophalangeal and extension of the proximal interphalangeal joints. Despite these deformities there is no pain, little functional disability and no joint destruction. Tests for rheumatoid factor are negative, the erythrocyte sedimentation rate is normal and there are no joint erosions.

The carditis is truly a pancarditis. Praecordial pain, a friction rub and S–T segment elevation signify a pericarditis. Tachycardia out of proportion to the fever, and cardiomegaly suggest a mycoarditis. This also causes E.C.G. abnormalities including prolongation of the P–R interval (more than 0.18 seconds in children under 15 is first degree heart block), arrythmias, prolongation of the QT interval and inversion of the T wave.

The endocarditis affects the mitral and aortic, more than the pulmonary and tricuspid valves, probably in proportion to the pressure gradients across each valve and to their respective degree of vascularity. The first effect of rheumatic fever on the valve is to cause it to contract towards its origin, thus valvular stenosis is not a feature of the first episode of rheumatic fever.

In the first episode of acute rheumatic fever, mitral incompetence may cause the soft first heart sound, systolic thrill and the classical blowing pansystolic murmur conducted into the axilla. More commonly, however, there is a less characteristic systolic murmur which may indicate increased flow across the normal valve, functional incompetence due to dilatation of the valve ring or may even by transmitted from the aortic or tricuspid valve. A rough ejection systolic murmur at the base transmitted into the neck indicates aortic valve stenosis.

In general diastolic murmurs are more significant than systolic murmurs. The mid-diastolic bruit which is quite frequently audible during the early episodes of rheumatic fever is called the

Carey Coombs murmur. The origin of this is disputed, but it may arise from left ventricular dilatation, and may either disappear during recovery or be superseded by the rough low pitched mid-diastolic murmur with presystolic accentuation, which indicates mitral stenosis.

Cardiomegaly with neck vein congestion and hepatomegaly in the early stages of acute rheumatic fever is often due to pericarditis with pericardial effusion, whereas later on it is more commonly due to congestive cardiac failure. Daily weighing is the best guide to fluid retention in children.

In patients with established rheumatic heart disease, sudden deterioration may be due to pulmonary thrombo-embolism, pulmonary infection, left ventricular failure which may have been precipitated by a rhythm change, subacute bacterial endocarditis or rupture of a valve cusp in addition to recurrence of rheumatic fever itself.

The histology of the heart lesions is distinctive. The Aschoff nodule occurs interstitially and comprises a central eosinophilic zone of 'fibrinoid' necrosis surround by a palisade zone of pleomorphic mononuclear and chronic inflammatory cells amongst which multinucleated giant cells are seen. Later fibroblast proliferation and fibrosis supervene. The Aschoff nodule is frequently related to small blood vessels and histological evidence of a proliferative or inflammatory vasculitis is usual. The valve cusps show oedema and neovascularization and later become fibrosed and contracted. Adherence of the leaflets leads to valvular stenosis. Chronic constrictive pericarditis does not follow the serous pericardial inflammation.

Subcutaneous nodules, which may occur in crops, vary in size from millimetres to centimetres and are to be found over joints, tendons and bony prominences. Histologically they are almost identical to the Aschoff nodule. They are distinguished from rheumatoid arthritis nodules by 'cropping', by their smaller size and by more rapid change in size. Histologically there is less pallisading and necrosis than in rheumatoid arthritis nodules.

Erythema marginatum is the typical dermatological manifestation of rheumatic fever, occurring in some 15 per cent of cases, and is almost pathognomonic of the disease. Transient red macular areas spread out in ring or map-like forms over the trunk and limbs sparing the face. Erythema marginatum may also very rarely be seen in drug allergy, trypanosomiasis or systemic lupus erythematosus. The typical skin rash of Still's disease is distinguished from erythema marginatum by the fact that it does not spread and that it is not 'ringed' with central pallor. Other skin manifestations of rheumatic fever which are less common include coincidental post streptococcal erythema nodosum or urticarial rashes.

A further, less common, manifestation of rheumatic fever which may occur in the absence of carditis or arthritis is Sydenham's chorea. This is a widespread meningo-encephalitis which begins insidiously with apparent 'clumsiness' and emotional lability. Characteristic purposeless, unco-ordinated, jerky spontaneous movements with pendular reflexes, ataxia and hypotonia are the features of the fully developed disease and in severe cases paralysis may supervene. Chronic valvular heart disease may follow chorea although there was no apparent cardiac involvement during the acute stage.

Serositis leading to abdominal pain may occur in acute rheumatic fever and acute streptococcal glomerulo-nephritis may follow the illness, occur with it, or even precede it. 'Rheumatic lung disease' is due to pulmonary oedema consequent upon congestive cardiac failure. Interestingly, subacute bacterial endocarditis rarely complicates acute rheumatic fever.

Laboratory Indices

A normochromic normocytic anaemia, polymorphonuclear leucocytosis and elevated erythrocyte sedimentation rate are common. There is usually evidence of recent streptococcal infection reflected in culture of the organism from the throat, or an elevation of the antistreptolysin O or antihyaluronidase titre. A rise in titre is particularly suggestive. The ASO titre may also be transiently elevated in Still's disease, tuberculosis and acute liver disease. Although the serum transaminase is not usually increased, lactate dehydrogenase levels may be markedly increased.

Treatment

Prophylactic treatment of streptococcal upper respiratory infections reduces the incidence of rheumatic fever. Although much is usually made of the difficulty of differentiating bacterial from viral throat infections, clinically there is much to be said for administering penicillin to all patients with upper respiratory infections provided the patient is not sensitive to the drug. This, however, will not abolish the disease entirely since many streptococcal infections are symptomless.

It is common practice to prescribe 2 weeks of oral penicillin to patients with acute rheumatic fever although this course is rather like shutting the stable door when the horse has bolted. The symptomatic treatment of choice in acute rheumatic fever is aspirin in a dose sufficient to maintain the serum salicylate level at approximately 30 mg per cent. This will dramatically relieve pain and will lower the temperature in the great majority of patients. Salicylism may occur insidiously since the therapeutic dose is close to the toxic dose. Occasionally aspirin may precipitate congestive cardiac failure. Corticosteroids (0.2 mg/kg/day) are indicated when the patient is gravely ill and in the presence of severe pericarditis or severe congestive cardiac failure. This must only be considered as adjunctive to the standard treatment of cardiac failure with diuretics, digoxin and oxygen and there is no evidence that corticosteroids affect the long term prognosis.

A great deal of discussion has been dedicated to the place of rest in acute rheumatic fever. Common sense rules should be applied to the individual case. Severely ill patients must be confined to bed, but unnecessary restriction of activity is not justified on the basis of one abnormal laboratory test.

Following recovery from the acute episode oral penicillin is given for 5 years, or until the age of 21. Some clinicians consider this to be inadequate and prescribe penicillin for much longer periods. Although recurrences do occur even with this precaution there is evidence that in the absence of penicillin the recurrence rate is very much greater.

Treatment of chorea is with bedrest and sedation. In severe cases hospitalization may be required. Penicillin prophylaxis should be given as for rheumatic fever.

Diagnosis

In a classical case the diagnosis of rheumatic fever is simple. The problem arises when only two or three of the manifestations are present. Arbitrary criteria (the Jones criteria) have been laid down which describe 'major' and 'minor' manifestations and allow some sort of score to be applied. This system is least reliable in precisely the cases where clinical doubt is greatest. In childhood, poliomyelitis, acute leukaemia, osteomyelitis, miliary tuberculosis, viral myocarditis, subacute bacterial endocarditis and appendicitis may cause confusion, but the greatest difficulty lies with Still's disease. In Still's disease the fever is remittent, the skin rash is typical and there is more lymphadenopathy. The cervical spine and sacroiliac joints are more frequently affected in Still's disease. Rheumatic fever is rare under 4 years of age, at which time Still's disease, Henoch Schonlein, purpura and leukaemia are more likely diagnoses of migratory polyarthritis. In the adult sero-negative rheumatoid arthritis or 'palindromic rheumatism' may cause confusion.

Prognosis

Severe carditis, a persistently high fever, and marked subcutaneous nodule formation denote a poor prognosis. If there is no evidence of carditis in the acute stage chronic valvulitis will follow in only 2 per cent of 'first episode' cases. It is extremely important to reassure these patients and their parents firmly. Typical auscultatory signs of mitral or aortic stenosis denote previous involvement and herald a worse prognosis. Over 70 per cent of these patients will have signs of established chronic valvular heart disease in later life.

Aetiology

Both the incidence and the severity of this disease are declining and there is some evidence to suggest that the incidence of chronic valvular rheumatic heart disease is beginning to decline also. Although much has been achieved in treatment and prevention, it seems likely that in this disease, like scarlet fever, there is a spontaneous trend inherent in the disease process which is as yet not understood.

There is now ample evidence implicating the Lancefield group A β-haemolytic streptococcus in the pathogenesis of acute rheumatic fever. Epidemiological evidence shows that the incidence of the disease follows that of streptococcal sore throats both seasonally, climatically and socially, both occurring in temperate climates, in poor social circumstances and in minor epidemics in closed communities such as military barracks. Serological evidence also indicates recent streptococcal infection which is usually in the upper respiratory tract, but may rarely be in wounds or even in the genital tract post partum. Furthermore, treatment of streptococcal infections reduces the incidence of the disease.

Equally clearly, however, the streptococcus alone does not cause the disease directly. Although many are infected, few develop rheumatic fever, and there is a latent period between streptococcal infection and the onset of the disease. Elegant experimental work has shown that cardiac muscle, and some strains of streptococci share an antigenic determinant. Antibodies formed to the organisms might therefore also damage the heart, and indeed gamma globulin and β1A complement have been demonstrated in the heart. It remains conceivable, however, that these antibodies are the result and not the cause of rheumatic fever although this is currently the most exciting development in the study of the aetiology of this disease.

Familial aggregation of rheumatic fever is easily discernable, but is probably produced by environmental factors. Poor housing, hygiene and nutrition with an attendant increased prevalence of streptococcal infections seem to be the most important factors in producing this. Further evidence against a major genetic factor in the aetiology of the disease is provided by lack of evidence of genetic linkage or of concordance in monozygotic twins.

Chapter 11

ANKYLOSING SPONDYLITIS, REITER'S DISEASE, PSORIATIC ARTHRITIS, BEHCET'S SYNDROME, ERYTHEMA NODOSUM ARTHRITIS AND ERYTHEMA MULTIFORME

ANKYLOSING SPONDYLITIS

Ankylosing spondylitis is a chronic inflammatory arthritis of the spinal diarthrodial and cartilaginous joints, which affects young males and which is characterized by a tendency to bony ankylosis of the affected joints.

Clinical Features (Fig. 27, Table 9)

The disease occurs in one to two per 1000 of the population, and males are affected about five times as frequently as females. The incidence is unaccountably much higher in certain ethnic groups such as the Haida Indians in British Columbia.

Early complaints such as low back stiffness or pain, and unusual discomfort after sitting for long periods, are insidious in onset and diagnosis is often delayed for many years. A history of pain or morning stiffness may often be elicited dating from adolescence.

In 10 per cent of cases the onset is in the peripheral joints particularly the hip or knee joint and rarely an acute onset simulating acute lumbar disc protrusion may occur.

Physical signs in the early stages may be absent. The first signs

Table 9 Ankylosing spondylitis

Low back pain/stiffness		Peripheral arthritis
Reduced thoracic excursion		Atlanto-axial subluxation
Bilateral sacro-iliitis	$\pm$	Iritis
Elevated E.S.R.		Aortitis
		Amyloid
		Fibrosing alveolitis

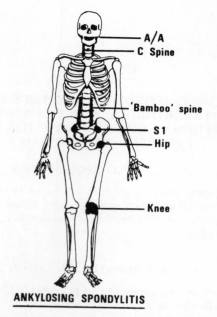

ANKYLOSING SPONDYLITIS

Fig. 27 Distribution of involvement in ankylosing spondylitis.

are of limitation of lateral flexion of the spine and paravertebral muscle spasm. Pain on compression of the pelvis or on backward pressure on the anterior superior iliac spines in the prone position should be sought although these signs depend on sacroiliac joint movement and are lost in the later stages when these joints fuse. Tenderness over bony prominences such as the trochanters and ischial tuberosities may be elicited.

In the later stages the physical signs are all too obvious. There is loss of all spinal movement and, improperly managed, the patient assumes the more comfortable, but more crippling attitude of flexion. There may be marked dorsal kyphosis. The cervical spine involvement is marked by the fixed flexed head, the patient having to rotate his entire body to see to the side and having to look upwards and bend backwards to see horizontally. It is particularly important at this stage to examine frequently for signs of hip involvement. The more rigid the patient's back becomes, the more does he rely on hip movement for locomotion.

Chest expansion may be reduced to less than 0.5 cm. Inguinal herniae may be present. A prostato-vesiculitis, sterile to conventional bacteriological methods, is present in a large proportion of patients, and is detected by examining the fluid following prostatic massage, when an elevated white cell count, and cell clumping, may be observed.

Systemic signs of severe disease include intermittent low grade fever, weight loss, a normochromic normocytic anaemia, and an elevated erythrocyte sedimentation rate (although this frequently is normal despite severe disease). The cerebro-spinal fluid protein level may be increased. Serological tests for rheumatoid factor are positive no more frequently than in the normal population and subcutaneous nodules do not occur.

The prognosis of ankylosing spondylitis has been variously assessed by different authorities as being better or worse than that of rheumatoid arthritis. Something of the order of one quarter of patients will become severely crippled and those with hip involvement tend to fare badly.

Pathology and Radiology

Early changes are in bone, particularly at ligamentous attachments, where a small focus of inflammatory osteitis develops. This invades the joint and neighbouring ligaments as granulation tissue grows in to be replaced by fibrous tissue and finally by cancellous bone. Similar changes are seen in the central cartilaginous and the central and peripheral diarthrodial joints.

The lymphocyte and plasma cell infiltrate, fibrosis and increased vascularity in synovium may be indistinguishable from rheumatoid arthritis. Erosions, narrowing of the joint space and peri-articular osteoporosis are seen on peripheral joint X-ray.

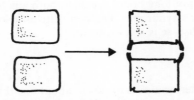

Fig. 28 Development from normal (left) of 'squaring' of vertebral bodies and of syndesmophytes.

In the spine the granulation tissue erodes the upper anterior margins of the vertebrae resulting in radiological 'squaring' of the vertebrae (Fig. 28) and grows out from the vertebral margins in the outer layers of the annulus fibrosus. When calcified the appearances of the later lesions are those of syndesmophytes which unite to form the 'bamboo spine'. This calcification is closely applied to the spine on X-ray differentiating it from other causes of paraspinal calcification such as Reiter's disease, psoriasis, paraplegia, Still's disease, fluorosis, ulcerative colitis, Crohn's disease, Whipple's disease, hypoparathyroidism, Baastrup's disease and familial hypophosphataemia in which calcification occurs in the longitudinal ligaments and is therefore separated from the spine by a narrow translucent band. Spondylitis may rarely antedate sacroiliitis in ankylosing spondylitis. The apophyseal joints are also frequently involved in ankylosing spondylitis.

The *sine qua non* for the radiological diagnosis of ankylosing spondylitis is *bilateral sacroiliitis*. Diagnosis may be difficult especially in early stages and the inter- and intra-observor error is high. Tomography may occasionally be of assistance but is usually the refuge of the uncertain. The early signs are of sub-articular increase in bone density alternating with osteoporosis and joint erosions which may give the appearance of widening of the joint. A radioisotope scan with radioactive strontium or fluorine may be abnormal before X-ray changes appear. In later stages the joints are completely ankylosed.

Bilateral sacroiliitis may occur in ankylosing spondylitis, Reiter's disease, Still's disease, psoriasis and paraplegia. Radiological changes are more commonly unilateral in all but ankylosing spondylitis and joint ankylosis is rare in these other conditions. 'Whiskery' fluffy exuberant periostitis of bony prominences such as the trochanters and the ischial tuberosities and of the ends of long bones occurs in both ankylosing spondylitis and Reiter's syndrome. The periostitis of psoriatic arthritis and of Still's disease is less exuberant.

Complications

Iritis. An anterior uveitis occurs in about one third of patients, but rarely leads to more than slight ocular discomfort. This is frequently unilateral and rarely it may be the presenting complaint. Young male patients with iritis should therefore be examined for the other features of ankylosing spondylitis. Very rarely glaucoma and blindness may be produced. Local installation of atropine and local corticosteroids are indicated. The association between uveitis, prostato-vesiculitis and sacroiliitis has been noted in Reiter's disease and in ankylosing spondylitis, but has never been explained.

The spine. Atlanto-axial subluxation occurs frequently and in association with the rigid brittle spine, this renders the patient extremely vulnerable to trauma. He should be cautioned about this and anaesthetists in particular must be aware of this possibility from the point of view of intubation. Long tract signs and quadriplegia may occur. Following even minor trauma fractures of the cervical spine are to be feared, but vertebral collapse lower down is less frequent than might be expected from the degree of osteoporosis, possibly because paraspinal ossification gives some degree of protection.

Heart. Isolated aortic incompetence occurs and the pathology resembles that of syphilitic aortitis. Thus the vasa vasorum are gradually occluded leading to focal medial degeneration and retraction of the valve ring. The valve itself is deformed, but because of the pathogenesis, aortic stenosis does not occur. Left ventricular hypertrophy, angina and interventricular conduction defects are also found. These complications are rare, occurring in only 5 per cent of patients, particularly in those with severe long-standing disease.

Lungs. An upper lobe fibrosing alveolitis has been described in ankylosing spondylitis. Maximum inspiratory flow rate is reduced, this being in contrast to the expiratory difficulty of emphysema. In general, however, the lungs remain surprisingly healthy in severe ankylosing spondylitis and respiratory function is less affected than might be expected possibly due to compensation by the diaphragm. The incidence of pulmonary tuberculosis and respiratory tract infections does not now appear to be increased as was formerly feared.

Amyloid is a rare complication of ankylosing spondylitis being of greater pathological interest than clinical relevance. The incidence of both ulcerative colitis and of regional enteritis is increased in patients with ankylosing spondylitis and conversely the incidence of ankylosing spondylitis is increased in these diseases. The reasons for these associations are obscure.

Diagnosis

This is simple in the presence of the classical presentation of spinal stiffness, reduced thoracic expansion, bilateral sacro-iliitis and a raised erythrocyte sedimentation rate. Difficulty is encountered when one of the complications, for example iritis, or peripheral joint involvement, is prominent at first, when the patient is female, and in the early stages when a young person complains only of low back discomfort. In all of these situations the diagnosis is made by thinking of it, by searching for the other features of the disease and if necessary by following the patient up. In certain rare instances the differential diagnosis between Reiter's syndrome and ankylosing spondylitis may be impossible at one point in time and may depend on follow up.

The other causes of sacroiliitis and paraspinal ossification present difficulty only from the radiological point of view.

Although paraspinal ossification in the longitudinal ligaments occurs in many conditions the co-existence of sacroiliitis excludes many of these such as fluorosis, idiopathic hypopara-thyroidism and Baastrup's disease. Baastrup's disease (senile ankylosing hyperostosis) is a disease of the elderly characterized by absent or mild clinical manifestations in the presence of florid dense calcification of both the anterior and lateral spinal ligament.

When sacroiliitis is bilateral, ankylosing spondylitis is the likely diagnosis since changes are more commonly unilateral in other arthritides such as Reiter's disease, Still's disease, psoriatic and rheumatoid arthritis infection and paraplegia. In ulcerative colitis, Crohn's disease and Whipple's disease the gastro-intestinal manifestations point to the diagnosis. Radiologically familial hypophosphataemia may be indistinguishable from ankylosing spondylitis, but the other features of the disease assist in differentiation.

It is important clinically to differentiate other causes of low back pain such as disc degeneration, spondylolisthesis, metabolic bone disease, trauma, Pott's disease, spinal brucellosis, primary or secondary spinal neoplasm, myeloma, and spinal osteo-chondritis (Scheuerman's disease), but again diagnosis is facili-tated by the other clinical and radiological features.

Treatment

The key to the management of ankylosing spondylitis is mobilization and in this disease physiotherapy has an important part to play. Although it may not always be possible to prevent progression it is usually possible to encourage ankylosis in an optimum position. This is achieved by frequent regular spinal and hip extension exercises which should be initiated by a qualified physiotherapist and continued on a regular basis by the patient. Immobilization of the patient during intercurrent illness is to be avoided whenever possible.

For mild disease salicylates are the drugs of choice in a dose of 3 to 5 grams per day. Patients may be controlled for many years with the above two simple measures. In the presence of progression, phenylbutazone (< 300 mg/day) or indomethacin (< 150 mg/day) should be prescribed. Rarely with severely afflicted patients low dose corticosteroid therapy may be required (< 10 mg/day). Synovectomy for an affected knee or replacement arthroplasty for a hip may be rewarding. Posterior spinal osteotomy may be considered in severe disease, but this technique carries with it an appreciable mortality.

Few would now advocate the use of radiotherapy which was previously employed without judicious control or assessment. Those who do respond to this would have responded to drug therapy. The incidence of aplastic anaemia and leukaemia in ankylosing spondylitis treated by radiotherapy exceeds the incidence in ankylosing spondylitis not so treated.

Aetiology

This remains unknown. This disease used to be considered a variant of rheumatoid arthritis. The sex ratio is, however, reversed; joint involvement is central in ankylosing spondylitis as opposed to peripheral, and even when rheumatoid arthritis does affect the sacroiliac joints involvement is usually asymmetrical. Subcutaneous nodules, peripheral neuropathy and arteritis do not occur in ankylosing spondylitis whereas iritis and aortic incompetence are not features of rheumatoid disease. Rheumatoid factor is present in ankylosing spondylitis no more frequently than in the general population.

Familial aggregation occurs in ankylosing spondylitis. No clearcut pattern of inheritance has emerged however, and the concept of autosomal dominance with reduced penetrance in the female has been rather tenuously invoked. It has recently been noted that the incidence of ankylosing spondylitis is increased in the male relatives of patients with Still's disease, and that patients with an initial diagnosis of Still's disease may later develop ankylosing spondylitis. The incidence of ankylosing spondylitis is also increased in the relatives of patients with psoriasis and Reiter's disease. The relevance of these observations has yet to be determined, but environmental factors have not been excluded.

On the basis of the high incidence of prostato vesiculitis it has been postulated that genito-urinary infection spreads via the pelvic lymphatics to produce the sacroiliitis. This possibility has similarly been invoked to account for the sacroiliitis of ulcerative colitis, regional iliitis and chronic paraplegic urinary infection.

REITER'S SYNDROME

Reiter's disease (Brodie's disease) is a disease of unknown aetiology characterized by urethritis, a sero-negative digoarthritis arthritis and conjunctivitis which affects young male patients.

Clinical Features (Fig. 29, Table 10)

This disease has a world-wide distribution and is by no means rare. Males are predominantly affected and the onset is usually between the ages of 20 and 40. Rare cases in females have been reported.

Table 10 Reiter's syndrome

Triad		
		Circinate balanitis
Urethritis		Keratodermia blenorrhagicum
Conjunctivitis	±	Prostatitis
Arthritis		Sacro-iliitis/periostitis
		Aortitis

Urethritis

This is the commonest of the triad and usually presents as a serous sterile urethral discharge with few clinical symptoms. Suprapubic discomfort, dysuria and haematuria when present,

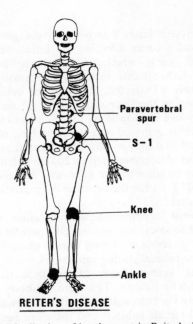

Paravertebral spur

S-1

Knee

Ankle

REITER'S DISEASE

Fig 29 Distribution of involvement in Reiter's disease.

are due to a haemorrhagic cystitis which may be detected by cystoscopy. Prostato-vesiculitis is extremely common and is detected either by examining the prostatic secretion after prostatic massage or by comparing five sequential specimens of urine for white cells. In the former test more than ten white cells per high power field is abnormal and in the latter there should be an excess of cells in the penultimate and last specimen. To be certain of the diagnosis it is preferable to have a large excess of cells and to see cell clumping. Apparently healthy young males may have a prostato vesiculitis by these criteria and so this test cannot be employed alone in the diagnosis of Reiter's disease.

Clinically it is extremely important to retract the patient's foreskin. Moist superficial ulcers may coalesce on the glans penis to form a circinate balanitis. The ulcers are painless thus differentiating them from herpes simplex. It should be routine practice to exclude both gonorrhoea and syphilis in the differential diagnosis of any urethritis in a young male.

Arthritis

This is characteristically a sero-negative asymmetrical oligo-arthritis of sudden onset affecting the knees, ankles or meta-tarsophalangeal joints which is subject to remissions and exacerbations. Other joints including the small joints of the hands may rarely be affected. Radiological evidence of sacro-iliitis is common in the later stages. Clinical manifestations of this are usually overshadowed by the symptoms in other joints. Pain in the heels is common and is caused by a plantar fasciitis.

Synovial fluid findings are non-specific, although large joint effusions are not uncommon. Up to 20,000 polymorphs may be found, viscosity parameters are abnormal and the glucose level may be reduced. Tests for the presence of circulating rheumatoid factor are negative.

Fever, elevated erythrocyte sedimentation rate, a poly-morphonuclear leucocytosis, non-specific protein changes and a normochromic anaemia are found during exacerbations, but all of these become normal during remissions.

A circulating auto-antibody to prostatic tissue has been detected in Reiter's disease. This auto-antibody has, however, alsc been detected in ankylosing spondylitis, in normal males and even in normal female subjects and therefore has no diagnostic value. Synovial membrane biopsy shows non-specific acute or chronic inflammatory changes with increased vascularity.

Radiologically, in the affected joints, para-articular erosions, narrowing of the joint space and peri-articular swelling are seen. Osteoporosis is less evident than in rheumatoid arthritis and periostitis of the metatarsophalangeal and the long bones is more exuberant and 'fluffy' than in rheumatoid arthritis. Plantar spurs also are more pronounced than in other diseases. A particularly characteristic finding is a single syndesmophyte arising from one vertebral body. Sacroiliitis may be very similar to that occurring in ankylosing spondylitis although it is more commonly unilateral in Reiter's disease. Psoriatic arthritis, Still's disease, Whipple's disease, ulcerative colitis, Crohn's disease infection and para-plegia may be associated with identical sacroiliac and para-vertebral radiological features.

Ocular involvement

Bilateral conjunctivitis with few clinical symptoms is the most frequent ocular manifestation of the disease. Culture is sterile by conventional bacteriological techniques. Rarely a painful unilateral or bilateral anterior uveitis may occur, especially in longstanding cases, but even then there are rarely lasting sequelae. Painful superficial keratitis and anterior synechiae leading to secondary glaucoma and blindness have been recorded. Conjunctivitis or iritis may precede the other signs of the disease and their occurrence in a young male should stimulate search and follow up to detect the other manifestations.

Mucocutaneous lesions

Apart from involvement of the glans penis and the urethra, painless shiny self-limiting lesions in the mouth may be confused with those of Behcet's syndrome, lichen planus, herpes, pemphigus and erythema multiforme. Pleuropneumonia like organisms have been isolated from the lesions, but their significance is not yet clear.

The typical, although uncommon skin lesion of Reiter's disease is keratodermia blenorrhagica, previously erroneously thought to be due to gonococcal infection. Initially macular, the lesions develop through yellow pustules to hyperkeratotic lesions on the palms and soles. These may persist for as long as 2 years, but usually disappear regardless of therapy. Florid destructive hyperkeratotic nail changes may occur.

Other features

Aortic incompetence similar to that of ankylosing spondylitis, pericarditis, and heart block are recognized complications of Reiter's disease.

Diagnosis

Where the complete triad of urethritis, seronegative arthritis, and conjunctivitis are present, diagnosis is simple. Syphilis and gonorrhoea may co-exist and should always be excluded. The features of gonococcal arthritis are described on page 141. Differential diagnosis of the individual features has been discussed. Particularly difficult presentations are that of acute febrile sero-negative polyarthritis in a young man in which case rheumatic fever and septic arthritis must be considered, and the late case with marked sacroiliac changes in which it may rarely be impossible to differentiate between Reiter's disease and ankylosing spondylitis. The speed of onset, pattern of development of clinical and radiological joint involvement, muco-cutaneous manifestations, greater tendency to develop large effusions, and lesser frequency of ankylosis in Reiter's disease will assist in differentiation.

Aetiology

In Europe the onset of Reiter's disease frequently follows a diarrhoeal illness, often of minor epidemic proportions whereas in the United Kingdom sexual exposure often antedates the disease. The time interval between those precipitating agents and the onset of the disease is highly variable. Neither are essential to the development either of the initial disease or the recurrences. The relationship between these precipitating factors and Reiter's disease has yet to be explained. A history of either, however, should stimulate a search for arthritis and conjunctivitis.

The clinical features of the disease suggest an infective aetiological basis. No pathogen has yet been causally related to Reiter's disease, however, despite numerous claims of isolation of spirochaetes, viruses, bedsonia and T strain mycoplasma. The agent under current investigation in Reiter's disease belongs to the bedsonia group and is similar to the trachoma virus. Isolation of this agent from synovial fluid has been reported, but remains to be confirmed. Bedsonia organisms (psittacosis-lymphogranuloma group) are intermediate in properties between bacteria and viruses.

Treatment

Joint. effusions are common and aspiration is frequently required to relieve discomfort. Local corticosteroid injections may be beneficial, but the dangers of repeated local injection must be borne in mind. Aspirin is the drug of choice and may be supplemented or succeeded by indomethacin or phenylbutazone. Rarely corticosteroid therapy may be required to control the symptoms. The indications for surgery in those rare cases which progress to joint destruction, are similar to those for rheumatoid arthritis.

Local corticosteroid applications may be required for the iritis but the conjunctivitis is usually self-limiting. The balanitis and keratodermia usually require only simple hygiene and the prevention of secondary infection.

In rare, severe cases methotrexate has been employed with benefit as assessed in a subjective uncontrolled manner. This toxic treatment must be reserved only for the most severe cases.

Course and Prognosis

Sequelae from the urethral lesions are very uncommon although stricture, renal infection and contracted bladder have been reported. Similarly both the ocular and skin lesions are commonly self-limiting. Recurrence of the arthritis has been assessed at 15 per cent per annum, but this is one of the more benign arthritides.

PSORIATIC ARTHRITIS

Psoriasis and rheumatoid arthritis are both common diseases each affecting approximately 2 per cent of the population. Clearly, therefore, these diseases will co-exist on occasions by chance alone. The incidence of 'classical' sero-positive rheumatoid arthritis is the same in psoriatic patients as in the general population. However, the incidence of sero-negative erosive polyarthritis is much greater in psoriasis than in the general population. This arthritis also shows distinctive differences from rheumatoid arthritis, particularly in the distal interphalangeal joint involvement, sacro-iliitis, better prognosis, equal sex incidence and the tendency of the severe form of the disease to undergo bony ankylosis.

The sero-negative erosive polyarthritis which occurs in patients with psoriasis, with a family history or past history of psoriasis, or with characteristic psoriatic nail changes is called psoriatic arthritis.

Clinical and Laboratory Features (Table 11)

Three patterns of arthritis are described although these are not mutually exclusive. There may be polyarthritis of insidious onset which characteristically involves the distal interphalangeal and sacroiliac joints and in which psoriatic nail changes are particularly common. Swelling may also be marked in the proximal interphalangeal producing an appearance known as the 'sausage' finger. 'Arthritis mutilans' is the least common, although most severe, expression of psoriatic arthritis. As the name suggests this is a deforming arthritis in which erosions and bone resorption may be marked. The typical radiological appearances are described as 'telescoping' of the phalanges and the 'opera glass' hand. The cervical spine, hips and sacroiliac joints are frequently involved. Finally psoriatic arthritis may occur as an arthritis which is clinically indistinguishable from sero-negative rheumatoid arthritis. These presentations should not be thought of as clearly delineated syndromes, but merely as guide lines to frequent clinical manifestations.

Rarely psoriatic arthritis may be present as an acute mono-articular arthritis. In association with hyperuricaemia, which occurs in 20 per cent of cases, this may trap the unwary into the diagnosis of gouty arthritis.

Table 11 Psoriatic arthritis

1. Family history or past history of psoriasis or the presence of psoriatic skin or nail changes
2. Sero-negative polyarthritis characteristically affecting the distal interphalangeal and sacroiliac in addition to other joints

Males and females are approximately equally affected although the mutilating form of arthritis is more commonly encountered in females. Non-specific features include normochromic normocytic anaemia, elevation of the erythrocyte sedimentation rate and hyperglobulinaemia. As with psoriasis uncomplicated by arthritis, intestinal malabsorption and elevation of the serum IgA level may be found.

Pathologically the features are of a chronic non-specific synovitis with oedema, increased cellularity, fibrosis and a lymphocyte and plasma cell infiltrate, which are not in themselves distinctive. An early feature common to both psoriasis and rheumatoid arthritis is capillary and venular dilatation and increased venular permeability, but the precise mechanism of these changes is not yet clear.

Radiologically para-articular erosions are particularly prominent in psoriatic arthritis giving rise to the 'pencil-cup' deformity of the terminal phalanges with 'whittling' of the middle phalanges (Fig. 30). However, this may also occur in rheumatoid arthritis and consequently the diagnosis cannot be made on this feature alone. Radiologically, the overlying psoriatic nail changes may be seen as calcification. Bony ankylosis of severely affected joints is a feature of psoriatic but not of sero-positive rheumatoid arthritis. Periostitis, especially in areas of muscle or tendon attachments is frequently seen.

Sacroiliitis occurs commonly, even in the absence of peripheral joint involvement, in patients with psoriasis and is usually asymmetrical. Paravertebral calcification may also be seen. The incidence of fully developed ankylosing spondylitis is higher than expected in psoriasis and in the relatives of patients with psoriasis. It would seem likely, therefore, that spondylitis and sacroiliitis should be considered as the fourth joint manifestation of psoriasis.

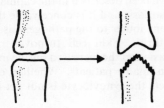

Fig. 30 Development from normal (left) of 'pencil-cup' deformity in psoriatic arthritis.

The skin lesions do not differ clinically or histologically from those of psoriasis without arthritis except for the higher frequency of nail involvement in psoriatic arthritis. This may take the form of 'pepperpot' pitting of the nail or, in its more severe forms, onycholysis. The nail bed may be inflamed and may simulate fungal or bacterial infection. Treatment of the skin lesions is along accepted dermatological lines. Parallel fluctuations of the skin and joint manifestations are unusual.

Aetiology and Pathogenesis

As is the case with psoriasis itself, the aetiology and pathogenesis of psoriatic arthritis are unknown. Familial aggregation of the disease occurs, but no definite Mendelian pattern of inheritance has been detected. Interest has been aroused by the familial aggregation and clinical overlap of psoriatic arthritis, Reiter's disease and ankylosing spondylitis. In all three there are certain common factors including sero-negativity, asymmetry of the polyarthritis, spondylitis or sacro-iliitis, a tendency to familial aggregation both individually and collectively, and non-specificity of the morphological features of the synovium. However, there are obvious clinical differences in the great majority of individual patients afflicted by each of these arthritides.

It has been suggested that trauma may induce in the psoriatic joint a process analogous to the 'Koebner' phenomenon in the skin. This is a tendency for psoriasis to occur in areas of skin which have been subjected to trauma. However, the pathogenesis of the 'Koebner' phenomenon itself remains to be elucidated. Abnormalities have been described in the capillaries in unaffected areas of skin in psoriasis and it is conceivable that a widespread capillary defect contributes to the pathogenesis of both psoriasis and psoriatic arthritis. Skin cell turnover rates are greatly increased in psoriasis and the increased purine metabolism causes hyperuricaemia in many patients. Whether or not the same phenomenon affects the synoviocyte is not yet known.

Treatment

Psoriatic arthritis is managed in accordance with the general principles of treatment of any chronic arthritis. It is best, however, to avoid the use of gold. Thus, although skin reactions are encountered in psoriatic patients no more frequently than in patients with rheumatoid arthritis treated with gold, it would seem wise to avoid the use of any compound which carries such a high risk of dermatological side effects where other treatment is available. Aspirin and non-steroidal anti-inflammatory compounds are usually sufficient to control the arthritis which tends to be more benign than rheumatoid arthritis. An exception to this is arthritis mutilans which usually progresses inexorably to joint destruction. Corticosteroids and synovectomy may be indicated in selected cases. Currently methotrexate and other antimitotic agents are being evaluated in severe psoriatic arthritis, but their formidable side effects demand that this treatment should only be prescribed in specialized centres. Early results with azathioprine however are encouraging. The indications for surgery in psoriatic arthritis are similar to those applicable to rheumatoid arthritis.

BEHCET'S SYNDROME

This clinical syndrome is characterized by three 'major' manifestations, namely, recurrent mouth and genital ulceration and iritis and many 'minor' manifestations the most frequent of which are; arthralgia or an asymmetrical sero-negative *oligoarthritis* in 60 per cent of cases; *septic skin* lesions in 30 per cent of cases; *vasculitis*; and *neurological* syndromes including optic neuritis, brain stem signs, a meningomyelitis or an organic confusional state with convulsions (Table 12). Less commonly erythema nodosum, thrombophlebitis, pericarditis and diarrhoea may occur. There may be fever, weight loss, hypergammaglobulinaemia and anaemia during exacerbations.

Table 12 Behcet's syndrome

Triad		
		Arthritis
Oral ulceration		Pyoderma
Genital ulceration	$\pm$	Neurological diseases
Iritis		Vasculitis
		Erythema nodosum
		Uveitis

Males are affected more frequently than females and the disease usually begins in the third decade. Clinical severity varies from remissions and exacerbations of symptoms of mild intensity to an acute fulminating fatal course dominated by central nervous system involvement.

Although a recurrent uveitis is the most common ophthalmological complication, keratitis, iridocyclitis with hypopyon, and intra-ocular thrombosis or haemorrhage may occur. The oral ulcers may be aphthous or herpetiform in type and the distinction is of some importance since the latter may respond to tetracycline. Vaginal ulceration presents as a purulent vaginal discharge and may cause severe dyspareunia. The arthritis commonly affects the knees or ankles, and synovial membrane biopsy reveals non-specific changes. Treatment of the arthritis with non-steroidal anti-inflammatory compounds is usually sufficient to control symptoms although synovectomy may be required.

The aetiology of this disease is unknown. Although an infective aetiology has been proposed, no organism has yet been causally related to the disease. Autoimmune factors are suggested by the presence of a circulating autoantibody to oral mucosa. This may simply be a 'marker' of the disease process. 'Allergic' factors have been proposed without any good evidence.

ERYTHEMA NODOSUM ARTHRITIS

The eruption is characterized by large, reddish-purple tender raised lesions on the shins which become discoloured and disappear gradually. They may appear in crops and may occur in any part of the limbs. An arthralgia of the knees and ankles is common, but occasionally there may be a frank synovitis and periarthritis with effusion which may persist for several months. The synovial fluid shows a polymorphonuclear leucocytosis. The prognosis even without treatment, however, is good.

Thrombophlebitis, cellulitis, chronic meningococcal septicaemia, nummular eczema, and nodular vasculitis due to polyarteritis nodosa, Henoch Schonlein purpura, Weber Christian disease or carcinoma of the pancreas may mimic the skin lesions, but the appearance of erythema nodosum is usually distinctive.

Although in many instances the cause is unknown, the following diseases are associated with erythema nodosum: tuberculosis, sarcoidosis, streptococcal infection, ulcerative colitis and Crohn's disease, drug allergy (these account for most of the cases occurring in Great Britain), leprosy, fungal diseases such as sporotrichosis, histoplasmosis, coccidiomycosis, toxoplasmosis and lymphogranuloma venereum.

Since many of these precipitating diseases are associated with abnormal delayed hypersensitivity responses and since no infective organism has been isolated from the lesion a cell mediated immune response abnormality has been proposed in erythema nodosum, but without confirmatory evidence to date. It is currently considered that the pathogenesis of erythema nodosum is that of an 'arthus' reaction.

ERYTHEMA MUTIFORME

This disease exists in two forms. In the benign and much more common form, the most prominent manifestation is an erythematous maculopopular rash which may be bullous in character and which particularly affects the distal limbs, and the mucous membranes of the mouth and eyes. Drug hypersensitivity (sulphonamides, phenobarbitone, phenylbutazone), mycoplasma pneumonia, herpes simplex and some foods and vaccines may cause this eruption which may be associated with fever and an acute self-limiting migratory polyarthritis. The syndrome usually disappears on withdrawal of the precipitant.

In the severe form (Stevens-Johnson syndrome), the rash is similar, but more widespread, and fluid loss from the ulcers may be marked. The arthritis is similar in distribution, but may be much more severe, at times even dominating the other clinical manifestations. To the skin rash and arthritis may be added renal failure, congestive cardiac failure or even a widespread bronchiolitis, any of which may be fatal. The precipitating factors in the Stevens-Johnson syndrome are the same as for erythema multiforme and it is not known why one patient may be severely, and another only mildly affected.

Chapter 12

GOUT

Gout is the clinical expression of an uncommon metabolic disorder characterized by hyperuricaemia and tissue deposition of monosodium urate crystals causing arthritis and renal impairment. The disease occurs predominantly in males.

Clinical Features

Acute gouty arthritis

This occurs suddenly, commonly overnight, in a middle-aged male. Precipitating agents include surgical operation, trauma, starvation diets, acute infections, and diuretic therapy. Individual patients may be able to associate the onset of acute gouty arthritis with many other factors including overindulgence in high purine foods or alcohol.

Characteristically, the first metatarsophalangeal joint is swollen, hot and excruciatingly painful. On rare occasions other joints may be involved leading to diagnostic confusion. The overlying skin is hot, dry, and purple in colour. Systemic manifestations include pyrexia, chills, anorexia, and elevated erythrocyte sedimentation rate and white cell count. In the absence of therapy, this episode usually settles completely in 1 to 2 weeks. A remission then follows which may indeed be of sufficient duration to allow the patient to outlive his disease. A patient has won an Olympic medal during this intercritical phase. More commonly, however, further episodes in this, and other joints, follow with diminishing time intervals and increasing residual joint damage.

Diagnostic clues to differentiate this from septic arthritis include a previous history of similar episodes with complete resolution, dry or desquamating as opposed to moist overlying skin, absence of lymphangitis or superficial abrasions, and the extreme severity of the pain in acute gouty arthritis. The presence of chronic gouty arthritis, tophi or renal impairment should be sought. The diagnosis is suggested by the raised serum uric acid and confirmed by finding monosodium urate crystals in aspirated synovial fluid.

Chronic tophaceous gout

Now that effective therapy is available this should become an increasingly rare phenomenon. Tophi occur in avascular areas on the helix of the ear, subcutaneously in relation to tendons or joints, or in juxta-articular bone. They consist of necrotic, pultaceous material surrounded by a zone of foreign body tissue reaction. Histologically the characteristic monosodium urate crystals can be seen in biopsy or aspirated material.

Radiological examination reveals the tophus as a radio-translucent clearly defined 'punched out' lesion in juxta-articular bone, which may form an erosion if placed peripherally. These erosions are more clearly defined than the erosions of rheumatoid arthritis and differentiation is further aided by cartilage preservation and by the relative lack of surrounding osteoporosis in gout. Other causes of juxta-articular cysts include osteoarthrosis, hyperparathyroidism, haemophilic and rheumatoid arthritis, sarcoid, myeloma, tuberculosis enchondromata and excessive work with the hands.

Important differential diagnoses of tophi on the ear include Darwinian tubercles (cartilaginous malformations which are translucent), basal cell carcinoma, and rheumatoid nodules. Subcutaneous tophi, particularly in relation to the elbow joint may also be mistaken for rheumatoid nodules, rheumatic fever nodules or xanthomata. Tophi related to nerves may rarely cause entrapment neuropathies.

Renal involvement

Monosodium urate crystals are deposited in the renal parenchyma and uric acid crystals in the tubules. A large proportion of gouty patients have minor degrees of renal involvement but hopefully, with increasing use of effective therapy, their numbers will diminish. It should be emphasized, however, that a number of untreated patients with chronic tophaceous gout will die in renal failure. About 17 per cent of patients with gout suffer from uric acid renal calculi. Acute uric acid lithiasis with anuria may complicate the early stages of treatment with antimitotic therapy in the myeloproliferative disorders.

The pathological features of the gouty kidney, in addition to reaction to crystal deposition in the pyramids, include accompanying vascular degenerative and hypertensive changes, and 'pyelonephritic' changes. It is helpful to assess renal function by creatinine clearance and intravenous pyelography at first attendance and to monitor thereafter by serum creatinine andurine protein analyses.

Rarely acute gouty arthritis or acute 'pseudogout' may complicate renal failure or renal dialysis. The rarity of overt clinical expression despite the frequent presence of high uric acid levels may be related to a diminished ability of uraemic patients to mount a foreign body reaction to the crystals.

'Secondary' gout

Secondary gout which is much less common than primary gout is the term used when there is an observable cause for the disease. The only difference between primary and secondary gout in clinical terms is the tendency for the serum uric acid to be much higher in secondary gout.

Although there are many cases of hyperuricaemia, all of which may occasionally be associated with gout (Table 12) very few of these factors are of clinical importance in causing gout. The great majority of patients with secondary gout have an underlying myeloproliferative disease, have taken one of the drugs which cause hyperuricaemia, or are undergoing starvation diets for obesity. Polycythaemia, usually of the primary variety, accounts for the largest numbers of patients with secondary gout in the first category. Approximately 8 per cent of these patients will develop gout. Diseases of the leucocyte and megakeryocyte are more liable to produce gout than are the diseases of the lymphocyte, probably because the cell turnover rate is higher and because these cells have a shorter life span than the lymphocyte.

Antimitotic drug therapy is becoming more widely used and consequently is accounting for more and more cases of gout. Allopurinol should be given prophylactically when the serum uric acid level begins to rise. Salicylates and diuretics may also cause secondary gout.

Diseases associated with gout

Hypertension, myocardial infarction, obesity and type IV hyperbetalipoproteinaemia are associated with a high incidence of gout, but the mechanisms of the inter-relationships is unknown. Gout is common in obese diabetic patients, but it seems likely that a major part of the relationship is with the obesity rather than the diabetes.

Treatment and Prognosis

Acute gouty arthritis

Although colchicine is commonly effective, particularly in the very early stages, the drugs of choice on the grounds of reliability, speed of action and relative lack of side effects, are phenylbutazone (800 mg per day for 3 days, reducing thereafter) or indomethacin (150 mg per day). Control of acute episodes in some chronic patients may rarely be extremely difficult requiring bedrest, analgesic and corticosteroid or ACTH therapy.

Chronic tophaceous gout

The decision to commence therapy, which should be continued for life, is taken in the light of the knowledge that on the one hand some patients may never suffer a second episode. On the other hand the probability of developing acute gouty arthritis is very high in the presence of a serum uric acid level persistently in excess of 9 mg/100 ml. Most physicians would now commence uricosuric or allopurinol treatment following the second episode or in the presence of marked overproduction. The decision not to treat should invoke as scrupulous follow-up as the decision to treat.

All patients must be instructed in the necessity of continued therapy and a high fluid intake. Alcohol excess, high purine foods and salicylates should be avoided. Weight reduction should never be precipitous.

The uric acid must be kept below 6 mg/100 ml. For uricosuric therapy probenecid is acceptable to most patients and has a low incidence of side effects, the most troublesome of which are gastro-intestinal. The dose of probenecid is approximately 2 to 3 g per day. The nephrotic syndrome, anaphylactoid skin reactions, status epilepticus and hepatic necrosis have been reported occasionally in association with probenecid and probenecid will potentiate the action of indomethacin. Sulphamethoxypyridine is used instead of probenecid by some clinicians.

Unequivocal indications for the exhibition of allopurinol include extensive tophaceous gout, renal impairment, antimitotic drug treatment and either intolerance or failure of response to uricosuric therapy. In the presence of demonstrable overproduction allopurinol is probably the drug of choice. Treatment should commence with a dose of 50 mg b.d. and the dose is then slowly increased until the serum uric acid is less than 6 mg per cent. Side effects include dyspepsia and skin rash, and white cell depression has been reported. The mode of action is discussed on page 133. The long term side effects of allopurinol are not yet known so the drug has not yet replaced probenecid in chronic gout.

In the early stages of uricosuric and of allopurinol therapy serum uric acid levels may fluctuate wildly, and acute gout is frequently precipitated. Accordingly concurrent therapy with oral colchicine (0.5 mg b.d.) is advisable. Oral colchicine may cause dyspepsia, diarrhoea, white cell depression, alopecia, and even death due to hypersensitivity. Serious side effects, however, are fortunately relatively uncommon. The mode of action, may involve the sol–gel transformation in the polymorph impeding motility and phagocytosis (Fig. 35), and so interrupting the inflammatory cycle.

The prognosis of a patient, properly managed following early diagnosis, is that of a normal life span.

Incidence

The incidence of hyperuricaemia and of gout varies widely throughout the world. Although only 50 of 3000 patients attending the Centre for Rheumatic Diseases in Glasgow have gout, in a population of New Zealand Maoris, 40 per cent of the males were found to be hyperuricaemic and 8 per cent suffered from gout. Females do not suffer from gout until after the menopause and then only rarely. Eunuchs and prepubertal males very rarely suffer from gout. These and many other fascinating observations remain to be explained. The increased incidence of gout in stressful occupations and in higher intelligence groups may be in part related to higher dietary purine intake. That this is unlikely to be the sole factor is suggested by the relative unimportance of exogenous as opposed to endogenous purines in uric acid metabolism.

Aetiology and Pathogenesis

To understand the aetiology and pathogenesis of gout it is first necessary to consider the normal and abnormal mechanisms of production and excretion of uric acid.

Uric acid is a $2:6:8$ trioxypurine, possessing two ionizable H^+ (pK_a 5.75 and 10.3). At pH 7.4 (body fluids) uric acid exists as a monovalent urate ion. Plasma saturation occurs at about 7 mg/100 and this explains why tophi do not resolve until the level of serum uric acid falls below this. Man lives with a serum uric acid level which is very close to saturation and it is surprising that gout is not more common. Albumin and other proteins are able to bind uric acid thus raising the amount which is required to saturate plasma, providing a possible explanation. In urine the pH is lower, and there is therefore more free uric acid.

Measurement of uric acid

Colorimetric methods exploit the ability of uric acid to reduce such substances as phosphotungstic acid with a resulting colour change. Other reducing substances such as ascorbic acid may be removed by alkalization and non-urate chromogens by storing. Caffeine salicylates and glucose will reduce phosphotungstic acid giving spuriously high values. Inter-laboratory variation is high and more recently the autoanalyser method has proved to be perfectly adequate for routine clinical purposes. The most accurate method utilizes the strong ultraviolet waveband of uric acid and its alteration as the uric acid is specifically digested by uricase. By this enzymatic spectrophotometric method the World Health Organization have defined the upper limit of normal as 7.0 mg for males and 6.0 mg for females. In population studies, uric acid levels are distributed unimodally about the mean. Occasionally therefore, normal subjects will be found to have levels in excess of those quoted, which represent two standard deviations above the mean value. This concept applies of course to many other biochemical parameters.

Before interpreting the results of serum and urine uric acid levels it is necessary to ensure that the patient was receiving no drugs which interfere with the production or renal handling of uric acid, and that renal function is not impaired.

Purine biosynthesis

The biosynthesis of the purines, adenine and guanine, provides structural material, energy transfer requirements and components of both DNA and RNA. Uric acid is produced by the degradation of these substances. The importance of endogenous as opposed to exogenous factors is underlined by the fact that a

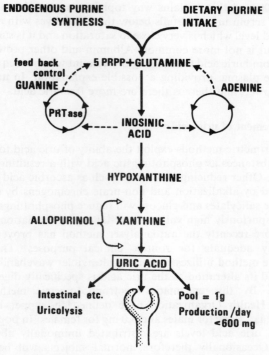

Fig. 31 Purine biosynthetic and degradative pathway.

purine free diet results in a reduction of less than 1 per cent in the serum uric acid.

The biosynthetic pathway is abbreviated in Figure 31. The rate limiting step, 5PRPP+glutamine, is under feedback control from below. Accordingly lack of an intermediary enzyme may result in gross overproduction of uric acid (Lesch-Nyhan syndrome). The compound allopurinol blocks the reactions hypoxanthine → xanthine and xanthine → uric acid. Serum and urine uric acid levels fall and xanthine and hypoxanthine levels rise. The latter are much more soluble in urine than is uric acid.

The miscible pool of uric acid is of the order of 1 g, daily production being rather less than this. Although uricolysis may occur in gut and in white cells, disposal is mainly by the kidney. The renal mechanism (Fig. 32) resembles that of potassium. All filtered uric acid is reabsorbed. Urinary uric acid derives from secretion by the tubules. This accounts for the paradoxical effect of salicylates and of diuretic drugs. Low doses block secretion

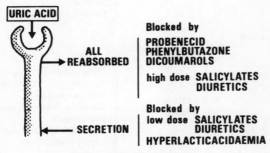

Fig. 32 Renal handling of uric acid.

and result in an increased serum uric acid whereas high doses paralyse both reabsorption and secretion and produce uricosuria. Individual variation is very high and therefore the net effect is too unpredictable to make these drugs useful in the management of gout. Other factors influencing the renal handling are shown in Figure 32. The inhibition of secretion by keto-acidosis may in part explain the hyperuricaemia of diabetic ketosis, starvation and glucose 6-phosphatase deficiency. The reabsorption transport mechanism is shared by other weak acids such as probenecid.

Provided the patient is receiving a purine free diet and is not receiving the above mentioned compounds, urine excretion of more than 600 mg in 24 hours indicates overproduction of uric acid. A figure of less than 600 mg does not, however, exclude overproduction. The ratio of uric acid to creatinine may be employed to diagnose gross overproduction of uric acid. Twenty-four hour values giving a ratio in excess of 0.68 indicate overproduction but ratios of less than this do not exclude it. These values are valid only in the presence of normal renal function.

Table 13 Hypo- and hyperuricaemia

Overproduction		
Familial	PRT deficiency	
	? Some cases 'primary' gout	
Acquired	Blood diseases Psoriasis Antimitotic drugs	Polycythaemia (1^y, 2^y) Myeloid, monocytic leukaemia Anaemias (especially P.A. treat with B_{12}) Myelofibrosis Myeloma Haemaglobinopathies
Undersecretion		
Familial	? Some cases 'primary' gout	
Acquired	Renal tubular impairment	Drugs (diuretics, aspirin) Acidosis (starvation diabetic ketosis alcohol) Uraemia, lead poisoning preclampsia Hypercalcuria (sarcoid hyperparathyroid)
Overproduction + undersecretion		Type 4 glycogen storage disease ? Some cases 'primary' gout
Undetermined		Down's syndrome Hypertension Acromegaly, myxoedema, hypoparathyroidism
Hypo-uricaemia		Pregnancy, hyperthyroidism Wilson's disease, Fanconi syndrome Acute intermittent porphyria Xanthinuria or allopurinol treatment

Hyperuricaemia

The various causes of hyperuricaemia are shown in Table 13. Hyperuricaemia is due to overproduction and/or undersecretion of uric acid. Only 25 per cent of hyperuricaemic patients will develop gout. The remainder live a normal lifespan with asymptomatic hyperuricaemia. The probability of developing gout is, however, closely linked to degree and 90 per cent of patients with a serum uric acid in excess of 9 mg/100 will develop gout.

Investigation of hyperuricaemia has been greatly aided by the application of radioactive tracers. The miscible pool and turnover rate can be simply determined by administering labelled uric acid intravenously. The slope of the graph A–B (Fig. 33) denotes the dilution of labelled uric acid by newly formed unlabelled uric acid

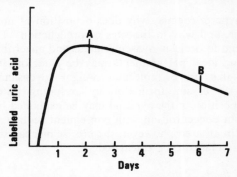

Fig. 33 Radioactive uric acid clearance curve.

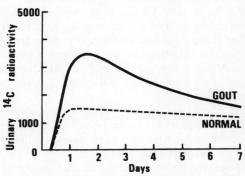

Fig. 34 Incorporation of ^{14}C-glycine into uric acid.

135

giving a measure of production. The presence of tophi renders this simple method invalid. However, the rate of incorporation of a labelled precursor (^{14}C-glycine) can then be employed and some gouty subjects demonstrate a greatly increased incorporation rate, showing overproduction (Fig. 34).

Only about 25 per cent of gouty patients can be shown to over-produce and many others possess a deficiency in the secretion of uric acid by the kidney. Many gouty subjects have a clearance of uric acid with respect of inulin which is reduced when compared with normal subjects at all levels of serum uric acid.

Crystal deposition

In tissue

Given hyperuricaemia, why does deposition of monosodium urate occur, and why in the sites of predeliction? Tophaceous deposits tend to occur in avascular areas and anaerobic metabolism causing local pH gradients may be a factor. It has been suggested that large molecular weight glycosaminoglycans predispose to crystal formation by excluding water. In the kidney, deposition in the pyramid may be explained by the high local sodium concentration with consequent reduction in urate solubility. In all areas, however, the precise mechanism of tissue deposition remains to be elucidated.

In synovial fluid

Mechanism of acute crystal deposition disease (gout and pseudogout). It is now known that deposition of uric acid crystals in synovial fluid causes acute gouty arthritis (Fig. 35). It is likely that the crystal size and shape is of more importance than its chemical constituents since a similar mechanism has been proposed for acute 'pseudogout'. Sodium orotate crystals and corticosteroid microcrystals of the same dimensions will also produce inflammation.

Following crystal deposition, polymorphonuclear leucocytes are attracted by chemotaxis to the crystal. Colchicine interrupts this stage of the cycle. Attempts to phagocytose the crystal may result in an increased production of lactic acid by the cell which then dies, releasing lysosomal enzymes and reducing local pH. Thereafter Hagemen factor, the complement system and the chemical mediators of inflammation may be activated resulting in the classical signs of the acute inflammatory response. Alteration in pH favours further crystal deposition completing the cycle. Precise physicochemical definition of those events is awaited but the concept seems likely to hold.

Identification of crystals

The demonstration of monosodium urate crystals is the only certain method for the diagnosis of gout. After evaporation to dryness with nitric acid, a purple colour will be produced when concentrated ammonium hydroxide is added if either urate or uric acid is present (Murexide Test). Positive identification is today accomplished either by observing dissolution on the addition of uricase, or by examination under the polarizing microscope. Monosodium urate crystals are negatively birefringent whereas calcium pyrophosphate crystals are weakly positive.

Genetics

Hyperuricaemia and gout are more common in relatives of gouty patients, the precise excess over a control population varying in different studies. The lack of agreement probably stems from selection bias and failure of uniformity in the method of uric acid assay. Recent evidence suggests that it is inappropriate to study the genetics of the 'gouty trait'. The delineation of incomplete and complete phosphoribosyltransferase (PRT-ase) deficiency (Lesch-Nyhan syndrome) which is transmitted as a sex-linked recessive trait has demonstrated that the gouty population is not a homogeneous group. It seems likely that many further discrete enzyme deficiencies exist which may each be transmitted differently. It is therefore to the individual family group that one should look for the elucidation of the genetics of gout.

PRT DEFICIENCY

The separate consideration of this extremely rare disease is justified by its illustrative role. It represents the first enzyme deficiency disorder to be discovered in gout. Clinically complete deficiency of the enzyme is expressed as choreo-athetosis, spasticity, mental retardation and auto-aggression. A macrocytic anaemia has been reported.

Absence of PRT results, either by loss of feedback control or by increase in available 5 PRPP, in gross overproduction of uric acid causing renal failure and gout.

Transmission would appear to be X linked but the patients do not live to produce so failure of transmission from male to male cannot be confirmed. It remains possible therefore that transmission is dominant with sex influenced expression. Fibroblast culture from mothers of affected children shows two cell lines (mosaicism); one cell line expresses the defect and the other is normal. This is in accord with the Lyon hypothesis the 'normal' cell having the abnormal gene on it's inactivated X chromosome (Barr body).

Incomplete PRT deficiency is expressed clinically as severe gout with only slight neurological signs. Gross overproduction of uric acid is present. Transmission from male to male does not occur, providing evidence of X linked transmission.

Treatment with allopurinol will usually control the hyperuricaemia, in PRT deficiency but will not affect the neurological features.

CHONDROCALCINOSIS OR 'PSEUDOGOUT'

Chondrocalcinosis is a clinical syndrome consisting of recurrent attacks of acute monoarticular arthritis, or more usually of chronic polyarthritis, in association with calcification in articular cartilage. The calcification, in the articular cartilage, is due to deposition of calcium pyrophosphate dihydrate crystals.

Clinical Features

The disease affects middle-aged and elderly patients. The knees are most commonly involved. A history of repeated gout-like attacks may be elicited, or a chronic form of arthritis may develop insidiously. X-ray of the knees, symphysis pubis, hip joints and wrists may show calcification of cartilage, these joints being most commonly affected. Aspiration of synovial fluid during the acute attack will reveal crystals of calcium pyrophosphate dihydrate, some of which may be inside polymorphonuclear leucocytes.

Cartilage calcification also occurs in ochronosis, haemachromatosis, Wilson's disease and hyperparathyroidism. Hydoxyapatite and dicalcium pyrophosphate crystals which are common in the elderly rarely cause symptoms although a periarthritis associated with hydroxyapatite has been described.

The erythrocyte sedimentation rate is normal, except during acute episodes. The serum calcium, phosphorus and alkaline phosphatase are normal in the absence of complicating hyperparathyroidism.

Diagnosis

Articular calcification is common in the middle-aged and elderly person and rarely leads to symptoms. The diagnosis of the acute attack rests on the demonstration of calcium pyrophosphate dihydrate crystals. Crystals of calcium pyrophosphate must be differentiated from other crystals in synovial fluid such as cholesterol or uric acid crystals, corticosteroid microcrystals, or orotic acid crystals which can be accomplished by X-ray diffraction patterns. When viewed under polarizing light calcium pyrophosphate crystals are positively birefringent whereas uric acid crystals are weakly negative.

Treatment

Treatment of the acute attack is similar to that of acute gout. Oral phenylbutazone or indomethacin and joint aspiration are beneficial in the acute stage. Chronic arthritis is managed symptomatically.

Aetiology and Pathogenesis

The cause of calcification in articular cartilage is unknown, but the acute attacks of arthritis are due to crystal-induced inflammation similar to that which occurs in gouty arthritis due to uric acid crystals (Fig. 35). It seems likely that the physicochemical properties of the crystals are of pathogenetic importance. Hyperparathyroidism and haemochromatosis may be complicated by chondrocalcinosis. A familial aggregation of chondrocalcinosis has been reported, but evidence as yet is lacking for predictable genetic transmission. It is of interest that artificial fertilizers contain calcium pyrophosphate, and conceivably ingestion of these may be a factor in the pathogenesis of the disease. Alkaline pyrophosphatase has been noted to be lower in the synovial fluid in this disease, but the relevance of this observation to the pathogenesis of the disease remains to be elucidated.

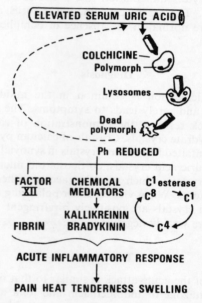

Fig. 35 Proposed self perpetuating pathway for crystal arthritis.

Chapter 13

INFECTIOUS ARTHRITIS

Septic arthritis

Septic arthritis may appear *de novo*, or may follow evidence of infection elsewhere. Predisposing factors include previous damage to the joint by disease or trauma, including operation or intra-articular injection, debilitating illness especially diabetes, and treatment with corticosteroids or with immuno-suppressive agents. Prematurity predisposes to infection of the hip joint with coliform organisms.

Usually there is an acute painful monoarthritis with a 'swinging' temperature, rigors and polymorphonuclear leucocytosis. The knees, wrists or elbows are most commonly affected although no joint is immune. Occasionally, especially with gonococcal infection, there may be a migratory asymmetrical polyarthritis. Gonococcal arthritis today is much more common in females than in males and tends to be chronic rather than acute. A history of sexual exposure is not often elicited. Clinical signs which should raise suspicion are rigors or chills, skin lesions and tenosynovitis. The disease will remit completely with penicillin. Salmonella arthritis is particularly common in children and usually affects the large joints. In acute meningococcal septicaemia, an acute polyarthritis or a purulent monoarthritis may be seen whereas in chronic meningococcal septicaemia a flitting migratory arthritis may accompany the other clinical manifestations which include fever, rigors and a petechial or maculopapular rash.

Differentiation of septic arthritis from trauma, osteomyelitis, gout, Still's disease or rheumatoid arthritis may be difficult on occasions and if there is any suspicion of sepsis it is mandatory to aspirate the joint when a purulent synovial fluid will be obtained. Identification of the organism and of its antibacterial sensitivity will determine treatment. The greatest diagnostic difficulty is encountered in established rheumatoid arthritis, particularly when the clinical signs are masked by corticosteroid treatment. Deterioration in one joint out of proportion to the others should suggest the diagnosis of septic arthritis.

It cannot be emphasized too strongly that delay in diagnosis, or inadequate treatment may have fatal consequences. Treatment is by repeated aspiration and local and systemic antibiotic therapy. Even with prompt treatment, septic arthritis super-vening upon a debilitated patient with rheumatoid arthritis carries a grave prognosis.

Tuberculosis

This is usually a subacute monoarthritis of the major weight bearing joints which may be remarkably painless. The patient usually presents with swelling of the joint which on clinical examination proves to be due to a combination of synovial hypertrophy and effusion. Onset is insidious, the history often extending over several months. Although any joint may be affected, it is the knees, hips and lumbar spine which are most commonly involved.

Today the joint is second only to the lung in the frequency of system involvement in tuberculosis. Although this used to be a disease of young adults it is occurring increasingly commonly in middle-aged or even elderly patients. Diagnosis is frequently long delayed, due partly to the insidious onset and partly to the altered age incidence, since it used to be thought of as a disease of young adults. Tenosynovitis and tuberculous dactylitis are rare today as too, is tracking of a 'cold' abscess to point in the groin.

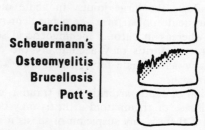

Carcinoma
Scheuermann's
Osteomyelitis
Brucellosis
Pott's

Fig. 36 Differential diagnosis of Pott's disease.

Radiologically there is soft tissue swelling, osteoporosis, cystic bone erosions which progress to marked bone destruction, and relative preservation of cartilage. When the vertebral body is affected (Pott's disease) there is marked bone lysis with vertebral collapse and loss of joint space. The appearances must be differentiated from Scheurman's disease, carcinoma, osteomyelitis and brucellosis (Fig. 36).

In the peripheral joints synovectomy is indicated for both diagnostic and therapeutic reasons. Treatment is with standard antituberculous chemotherapy and immobilization. Surgical intervention, other than synovectomy, is less commonly required today than formerly.

Brucellosis

Arthritis is a common manifestation of brucellosis, a disease which is endemic in this country. In some countries which have more advanced public health programmes, brucellosis has been eradicated. The 'abortus' type is the one most commonly encountered in the United Kingdom. There is intermittent fever, weight loss, sweating and a history of exposure to farm animals and their produce will be elicited. An arthralgia or a mild and self-limiting arthritis of the shoulders, knees and elbows are the most common articular manifestations.

A destructive subacute arthritis of the hip or knee, and sacroiliitis or spondylitis may occur and in some patients the spondylitis may even dominate the other clinical features. The upper anterior vertebral margin is eroded and spur formation is characteristic. A rise in brucella agglutinin titre is the best method of diagnosing the disease since blood cultures are rarely positive and skin testing is unreliable. Treatment is with tetracycline and streptomycin.

In *leprosy*, atrophic arthritis, Charcot's joints and immobilizing contractures may occur due to peripheral neuritis. Erythema nodosum with arthritis of the knees and ankles may complicate treatment with sulphones. Very rarely an acute peripheral polyarthritis may occur during the course of the disease itself.

Viral Infections

An acute, self-limiting polyarthritis and tenosynovitis may complicate *rubella* and an absence of polymorphonuclear cells with an increase in mononuclear cells, provides a distinctive synovial fluid picture. This arthritis is particularly common in young adult female patients In *mumps*, which is particularly common in adult males, an oligo- or monoarthritis of the elbow, ankle or less commonly the joints of the hands may occur in the second week of the disease. Arthritis occurs in *smallpox*, but is overshadowed by the other clinical manifestations.

The major importance, from the rheumatological point of view, of the arthralgia which may occur in *infectious mononucleosis* lies in the possibility of confusing it with acute rheumatic fever, or Still's disease. The arthritis of *lymphogranuloma venereum* affects the lower limb joints and is usually chronic although an acute migratory arthritis may occur. The Frei skin test is positive. *Arbor 'A' viruses* of epidemic polyarthritis, Chikungunya and O'Nyong-Nyong fever may cause an excruciatingly painful polyarthritis which may persist for many months.

Spirochaetal Diseases

Yaws, which can be differentiated from syphilis only by a negative treponema immobilizing test since the Wasserman reaction is positive in both, is characterized by bony rather than articular disease.

In acquired syphylis, bone and joint gummata, intermittent hydrarthrosis of the knee joints, periostitis and Charcot's joints may occur. A flitting polyarthritis may accompany the skin eruption of the secondary stage. In congenital syphylis, epiphysitis and osteochondritis are more common than arthritis. Chronic intermittent hydrathrosis (Clutton's joints) may occur in adolescents with congenital syphylis in association with eighth nerve deafness, interstitial keratitis and Hutchison's teeth.

Fungal Diseases

Fungal infection of the joints is common in many parts of the world, but is rare in the United Kingdom. Patients who develop one of these diseases in Britain are usually those who are receiving high dose corticosteroid therapy, radiotherapy, immuno-suppressive therapy or antibiotics. Infection may occur by contact with soil or dust, by inhalation, or by direct inoculation. Clinically the presentation is similar to that of a septic arthritis and in most of the fungal diseases osseous, cutaneous or pulmonary infection overshadows the articular manifestations. Eosinophilia and erythema nodosum may occur.

Diagnosis is by direct demonstration of the fungus in aspirated material or by a rise in circulating antifungal antibodies. Positive skin tests are only of value in histoplasmosis and coccidiomycosis and even then only indicate either past or present infection. Treatment with penicillin is effective only in actinomycosis. Either amphoteracin B or 2-hydroxystilbamidine are required in cryptomycosis, histoplasmosis, blastomycosis, coccidiomycosis aspergillosis, and sporotrichosis.

Chapter 14

ARTHRITIS ASSOCIATED WITH GENERAL
MEDICAL DISEASES

Blood Diseases

Haemophiliac arthritis

The most crippling complication of haemophilia is arthritis. This occurs in those haemophiliacs who are severely affected, with levels of antihaemophiliac globulin of less than 2 per cent, and onset is usually in childhood. The knee and the elbows are most frequently affected. Either spontaneously or after very minor trauma the joint becomes swollen and there may be local tenderness and warmth of the overlying skin. Joint mobility, commonly preserved during the first episode, is progressively lost with further episodes and severe joint deformity and destruction ensue. Extra-articular musculo-skeletal complications due to bleeding into soft tissue include compression neuropathies and Volkmann's ischaemic contracture.

Pathologically there is a chronic non-specific synovitis with extensive haemosiderin deposition and fibrosis. Minute haemorrhages occur both in the joint and in underlying juxta-articular bone. Radiologically severe juxta-articular osteoporosis and large subchondrial bone cysts, which are particularly suggestive of haemophiliac arthritis, are seen in the early stages. Later cartilage destruction is expressed radiologically as loss of joint space, and severe secondary osteoarthrosis and joint destruction may develop. Fibrous ankylosis may occur, but bony ankylosis is uncommon. Additional radiological features include 'squaring' of the patella due to flattening of its lower pole, epiphyseal dysgenesis or premature closure, and periosteal elevation with subperiosteal haemorrhage and calcification in the shafts of the long bones which may require differentiation from bone tumour.

Treatment of the acute episode is to arrest bleeding as quickly as possible with fresh frozen plasma or with cryoprecipitate if available. The joint should be·immobilized, surrounded by ice packs and as soon as the haemostatic defect is corrected aspiration with a wide bore needle helps to prevent irreversible changes from developing. Mobilization should begin as quickly as possible. Orthopaedic measures for the relief of chronic deformities are becoming increasingly successful, but require to be 'covered' by fresh frozen plasma or cryoprecipitate. Prophylactic advice should be offered to all haemophiliac patients as a routine with particular reference to avoidance of trauma. However, the youth of so many of the patients and the small amount of trauma required to produce bleeding restrict the value of this.

The articular manifestations of Christmas disease are similar to those of haemophiliac arthritis in all but treatment. It is not necessary to use fresh frozen plasma since reconstituted dried plasma will correct the haemostatic defect in Christmas disease.

Sickle cell disease

Arthralgia is common in sickle cell disease, and is usually expressed as painful swelling of the hands and feet, and backache. The pathogenesis is complex. Thrombosis with multiple infarctions occurs in small bone blood vessels due to sickling of the erythrocytes during hypoxia, and there is extension of haemopoetic marrow into the vertebrae and long bones compensatory to severe anaemia.

Radiologically, multiple bone cysts, cortical thinning, osteoporosis of the vertebrae, periosteal elevation in the metacarpal and metatarsal shafts, and the 'hair on end' appearance of the skull due to thickening of the calvarium may be seen. Thrombosis of a large vessel may result in aseptic necrosis of an entire epiphysis.

Leukaemia, myeloma and the reticuloses

Bone pain is a frequent presenting complaint in myeloma and is more common in leukaemia than is pain in the joint. However, a migratory polyarthritis accompanied by fever which resembles rheumatic fever may herald the onset of leukaemia in childhood. Associations between the lymphomas and hypertrophic pulmonary osteoarthropathy, rheumatoid arthritis, systemic lupus erythematosus, and Sjøgren's syndrome have been documented.

Rarely myeloma may be associated with either a symmetrical rheumatoid-like polyarthritis or an oligo-arthritis with marked synovial hypertrophy and pericollagenous amyloid deposition. Myeloma is suggested by a very high erythrocyte sedimentation rate, renal impairment and urinary Bence-Jones protein.

Secondary gout may complicate polycythaemia, acute leukaemia, myeloma, the malignant lymphomas and chronic myeloid but not lymphatic leukaemia.

Agammaglobulinaemia

This may be congenital or acquired and may be associated with impaired cell mediated immune responses. An arthritis clinically almost indistinguishable from rheumatoid arthritis or Still's disease is present in about one third of patients. The erythrocyte sedimentation rate is normal, rheumatoid factor is absent from the peripheral blood and there are no plasma cells in the synovium. Subcutaneous nodules and joint erosions, however, are common. The distribution of the arthritis tends to be less symmetrical than in rheumatoid arthritis. Systemic lupus erythematosus, scleroderma and dermatomyositis have also been recorded in patients with agammaglobulinaemia.

Haemachromatosis

Arthritis frequently complicates, and rarely may antedate the appearance of haemachromatosis. In some cases the arthritis has all the features of pseudogout. Clinically there may be acute episodes of joint pain, tenderness and swelling, or a chronic arthritis. Crystals of calcium pyrophosphate dihydrate may be aspirated or demonstrated in cartilage at autopsy and intra-articular calcification of the wrists, knees or symphysis pubis may be seen on radiological examination.

In other patients there are no calcium pyrophosphate crystals and the pathogenesis is unknown. The joints of the hands and wrists may be involved alone, or the hips, knees and shoulders may also be involved.

Radiological features include loss of joint space, juxta-articular osteoporosis, cyst formation and subarticular sclerosis mimicking osteoarthrosis. Osteophytes however, are less prominent than in osteoarthrosis. The pathogenesis and inter-relationships of haemachromatosis, pseudogout and haema-chromatotic arthritis require further study.

Gastro-Intestinal Diseases

Ulcerative colitis and Crohn's disease

The two articular manifestations of both ulcerative colitis and regional ileitis are remarkably similar despite the other clinical and immunological differences between these diseases.

Firstly a peripheral inflammatory arthritis may commence in one joint, but usually spreads to involve the small joints of the hands and the knees in a symmetrical fashion. The arthritis may be migratory and may fluctuate with the course of the gastro-intestinal disease, but is usually benign. The only difference between this arthritis in the two diseases is that the proximal interphalangeal joints are involved commonly in Crohn's disease and uncommonly in ulcerative colitis.

Secondly classical ankylosing spondylitis may occur in both diseases. This differs in no way from ankylosing spondylitis in the absence of inflammatory bowel disease except that the male predominance in prevalance is less marked. The relationship between the bowel and joint diseases is most marked and is bi-directional in the case of patients with ulcerative colitis. In ulcerative colitis, sacro-iliitis occurs in 20 per cent of cases in the absence of other features of ankylosing spondylitis and may be associated with anterior uveitis.

Whipple's disease

This rare, potentially fatal disorder is more common in males than in females and is characterized by recurrent fever, steator-rhoea, hypotension, pigmentation, polyserositis, lymphadeno-pathy and polyarthritis. The arthritis is a major manifestation and is usually symmetrical. The course may be migratory and the large joints are affected, particularly the knees, shoulders and wrists. Sacro-iliitis may be seen radiologically. The aetiology is unknown, but treatment with a broad spectrum antibiotic may be effective. Recent description of inclusion bodies in macro-phages of the gut raises the possibility of infection in the aetiology

149

of this disease. The infectious agent currently implicated is a corynebacterium.

Hepatic disease

An inflammatory polyarthritis may complicate infectious hepatitis and Laennec's cirrhosis and may indeed be the presenting complaint. In these diseases the arthritis is usually benign and self-limiting. Biliary cirrhosis may occur in Sjøgren's syndrome. Lupoid hepatitis is described elsewhere.

Endocrine Disorders

Parathyroid disease

Patients with hyperparathyroidism frequently complain of bone pain and of vague arthralgia. Crush lesions and collapse of porotic cystic juxta-articular bone may produce a traumatic synovitis, particularly in the knee joints, which may be very severe and may be followed by the development of secondary osteoarthritis. Both gout and pseudogout may be associated with hyperparathyroidism.

Radiological changes of hyperparathyroidism include sub-periosteal bone resorption particularly of the phalanges and the inferior border of the pubic arch; generalized osteoporosis; bone cysts in the mandible, metacarpals, pelvis and clavicles; osteoclastoma; juxta epiphyseal bony sclerosis in children, and osteosclerosis in the 'rugger jersey' spine in hyperparathyroidism secondary to renal failure.

In idiopathic hypoparathyroidism paraspinal calcification in the lateral longitudinal ligaments may cause confusion with ankylosing spondylitis radiologically, but the other features clearly separate the diseases.

Acromegaly

Arthralgia is a common accompaniment of acromegaly. There may be abnormal mobility of joints due to soft tissue enlargement, and remodelling of the heads of the long bones and phalanges may be marked. The phalangeal shafts are thin and osteoporotic. Synovial and periarticular tissue proliferates and

150

the articular cartilage also hypertrophies producing increase in joint space radiologically. In addition to bony remodelling, consequent upon the alteration in the congruity of the articulating surfaces, osteophytes appear and typical 'tufting' of the terminal phalanges may be seen radiologically.

Thyroid disease

In juvenile hypothyroidism, epiphyseal dysgenesis and delay in epiphyseal closure are reliable diagnostic features. In adult hypothyroidism, arthralgia and generalized musculo-skeletal symptoms must be differentiated from hypothyroid myopathy. The carpal tunnel syndrome may occur in hypothyroidism. Both hyperuricaemia and gouty arthritis may also occur. A rare and late manifestation of hyperthyroidism, thyroid acropachy, is associated with exophthalmos and pretibial myxoedema. There is clubbing of the fingers and toes and periostitis particularly of the phalanges and metacarpals. This is exuberant and tends to be denser than that of hypertrophic pulmonary osteoarthropathy but rarely extends to the long bones of the limbs.

Diabetes

A Charcot's joint of the lower limb may develop in a patient with diabetic neuropathy. The incidence of osteoarthrosis of the knees and of peri-articular calcification is elevated in diabetic patients.

Diseases of the Nervous System

The protective influence of paralysis of a limb on the development of rheumatoid and of osteoarthrosis has been described.

Charcot's joints

Massive joint destruction and instability may develop insidiously and painlessly, but there may be recurrent swelling and rarely in the early stages the joint may be the seat of recurrent painful episodes characterized by all of the signs of acute inflammation. In syringomyelia the upper limb joints are affected and in tabes dorsalis or diabetes it is the lower limb joints which bear the brunt of the disease. Other rare causes include spinal nerve root damage, leprosy, subacute combined degeneration of the cord, spina bifida, repeated local injections of corticosteroid drugs and congenital insensitivity to pain.

Radiologically there are both destructive and hypertrophic changes with remodelling and osteophytosis. Joint instability is the predominant clinical finding. Pyogenic infection, haemorrhage, pressure neuropathy of nerves related to the joint, fractures of adjacent bone and dislocation may occur.

Renal Diseases

Joint effusions, particularly of the knees, may occur during the anasarca of renal failure. Gout, pseudogout and the arthritis of secondary hyperparathyroidism may occur both in renal failure and following renal transplantation. Calcium apatate crystal synovitis and an as yet uncharacterized acute asymmetrical polyarthritis may also occur.

Hypertrophic pulmonary osteoarthropathy

This is essentially a chronic periostitis affecting the distal limb long bones at the wrists and ankles associated with clubbing of the fingers and a non-destructive, non-specific, acute recurrent synovitis of large joints. Treatment is that of the underlying disease which is usually a primary pulmonary or gastric neoplasm or cirrhosis. Abnormal peripheral circulatory reflex control may be involved in the pathogenesis of the disease. Although clubbing may occur in the absence of hypertrophic pulmonary osteoarthropathy the converse is not true.

In clubbing there is loss of the obtuse angle at the nail bed, proliferation and increased vascularity of the soft tissues at the nail bed which may impart a warm fluctuant feeling on palpation, longitudinal nail striations, and increased curvature of the nail in both planes. The aetiology is unknown and clubbing may be seen in a wide variety of diseases including carcinoma of bronchus, the mediastinum, and the upper respiratory tract; pulmonary metastases; Hodgkin's disease; septic lung disease and hydatid lung cysts; subacute bacterial endocarditis and cyanotic congenital heart disease; liver disease including biliary and portal cirrhosis; diarrhoeal illnesses including ulcerative colitis and regional enteritis; syringomyelia, arteriovenous aneurism and myeloid leukaemia.

Pachydermo-periostitis is a condition which occurs in young males. There may be a family history. The joints are never swollen or tender, there is no relationship to underlying disease, and the periostitis is usually thicker and denser than in hypertrophic pulmonary osteoarthropathy.

In thyroid acropachy the periostitis is irregular and exuberant and affects the phalanges more than the distal ends of the long bones.

Sarcoid

Arthritis may be a major manifestation in sarcoidosis and may indeed precede the other features of the disease. It is useful to consider arthritis in sarcoidosis as being of two kinds. The first is acute in onset and carries a good prognosis. The second is chronic, occurs in established disease usually associated with evidence of sarcoid in other organs, and carries a poor prognosis. In the former the onset is acute and polyarticular, the peripheral joints in the hands and feet and the knees bearing the brunt of the disease. Recurrent episodes of 3 to 6 weeks duration may occur, but in some patients there may be only one episode.

The chronic destructive arthritis is more common in Negroes and is usually accompanied by other signs of sarcoid such as chronic uveitis and skin, hepatic and pulmonary involvement. Eosinophilia, hypercalcaemia, hyperuricaemia and hyperglobulinaemia may occur, and tests for rheumatoid factor are positive more frequently than expected. The tuberculin test is often negative reflecting a widespread impairment of the cell mediated immune response which occurs in sarcoidosis. The Kveim skin test, using an antigen prepared from a spleen which was affected by sarcoid, may be positive, but a negative result does not exclude the diagnosis. Synovial membrane biopsy may show only a chronic non-specific synovitis, but on occasions may reveal granulomata which may be characteristic but are never diagnostic. Radiological changes appear late and are therefore of limited diagnostic value. The joint space is narrowed and mottled rarefactions and multiple 'punched out' cystic areas may be seen in the metacarpals and phalanges.

'Punched out' lesions also occur in gout, osteoarthrosis, haemophilia, rheumatoid arthritis, hyperparathyroidism, enchondromatosis, polyostotic fibrous dysplasia, multiple myeloma, leprosy and systemic fungal disease.

Acute sarcoidosis in adolescents and young adults presenting with high fever, polyarthritis, hilar adenopathy, uveitis and parotitis responds well to symptomatic treatment and carries an excellent prognosis. Chronic sarcoid arthritis is also managed symptomatically, but carries much more serious prognosis.

Metabolic Diseases

Marfan's syndrome (homocystinuria, Ehlers Danlos syndrome)

These patients are tall, with elongated extremeties and the most frequent abnormalities are arachnoidactyly, high arched palate, ectopia lentis and musculo-skeletal abnormalities such as ligamentous laxity, talipes equinovarus and kyphoscoliosis. The connective tissue of the heart and aorta may be diseased leading to dissecting aortic aneurism, aortic incompetence or heart block. Other ophthalmological defects, include blue sclera, pupillary abnormalities and retinal detachment.

Recurrent painful joint effusions may occur, presumably related to the ligamentous laxity, and low back pain with sacro-iliac sclerosis and kyphoscoliosis may occur together and require differentiation from ankylosing spondylitis. Marfan's syndrome may also be confused with Achard's syndrome in which there is arachnoidactyly, ligamentous laxity and micrognathia.

Ectopia lentis, dissecting aortic aneurism and skeletal abnormalities also occur in association with mental retardation and thrombo-embolic phenomena due to an inherited deficiency of cystathionine synthetase in homocystinuria. There is a failure of conversion of homocysteine and serine to cystathionine in this disease. Homocysteine is oxidized to homocystine and also reconverted to methionine. The elevated urinary values of these amino acids confirms the diagnosis. It is important to diagnose this disease since a low methionine diet may be clinically beneficial. Interestingly some patients with Marfan's syndrome have elevated homocystine levels in their urine raising the possibility that this too is an inborn error of methionine metabolism.

In the Ehlers Danlos syndrome, joint hypermobility, blue

sclera, kyphoscoliosis and dissecting aneurism may occur, simulating Marfan's syndrome and both Marfan's and the Ehlers Danlos syndrome may occur in the same family. However, the extreme elasticity, atrophy and bruising of the skin in the Ehlers Danlos syndrome provides a distinctive difference.

Radiologically, the metacarpal index gives a quantitative expression of arachnoidactyly by relating the length to the width of the metacarpals. Values over eight, indicate arachnoidactyly, but a normal value does not exclude the diagnosis of Marfan's syndrome if sufficient of the other clinical signs are present.

Ochronosis (alkaptonuria)

This autosomal recessive disorder is characterized by dark pigmentation of skin and cartilage and by arthritis. The enzyme homogentisic acid oxidase which converts homogentisic acid to mallylacetoacetic acid is absent, and the urine and tissues contain an excess of homogentisic acid and its precursors. The urine turns black on standing or with alkalinization and black renal calculi may occur. Both sweat and cerumen are black and deafness may develop.

The arthritis, however, is the major manifestation, and varies in severity from a mild arthralgia to a severe crippling arthritis of the spine and large joints particularly of the lower limb. Onset is unusual before middle age. Pigmentation of cartilage and intervertebral discs (ochronosis) precedes tissue destruction which occurs by a mechanism which has yet to be defined. Radiologically narrowing of the intervertebral disc spaces, sclerosis, eburnation and osteophytosis may be seen and analogous changes occur in the peripheral joints. The shoulder is so rarely the seat of marked osteophytosis that its occurrence in that site should suggest ochronosis or pseudogout.

The urinary discolouration is distinguished from that of porphyria, bile pigments, melanoma, intravascular haemolysis and drug induced discolouration by the high homogentisic acid content. Very rarely resorcinol or hydroquinone may induce ochronosis in normal persons. Treatment of ochronosis is symptomatic, but if started early a tyrosine and phenylalanine free diet may be of value. Avoidance of consanguinous marriage will reduce the incidence of this disease.

Mucopolysaccharidoses

The clinical manifestations of this group of very rare diseases usually appear in the first 2 years of life and include mental and physical retardation, skeletal abnormalities and defects of connective tissue in viscera especially the eye, aorta, liver and spleen. All are transmitted as autosomal recessive diseases with the exception of Hurler's syndrome in which transmission is sex-linked and recessive. It seems likely that all are due to specific enzyme defects in the formation of the glycosaminoglycan component of connective tissue with excess urinary excretion of a precursor. The possible role of integrity of the lysosomal membrane in these diseases, as in the lipodystrophies is currently being studied.

Hurler's syndrome (gargoylism) is the most common of the group. Blindness due to either corneal opacity or retinal detachment, mental and growth retardation, hepatosplenomegaly and gross characteristic skeletal abnormalities appear in infancy. The skull is large, the nose flat, the lips enlarged and the skin is coarse. There is hyperteleorism, talipes equinovarus, coxa valga and clawing of the fingers and toes due to loss of elasticity in peri-articular tissue. The phalanges are short, broad and malformed and vertebral body collapse may be seen. Metachromatic granules may be demonstrated in polymorphonuclear leucocytes or bone marrow and the urinary concentration of chondroitin sulphate B and hepartin sulphate is elevated. Many patients die in cardiac failure due to a chronic endocarditis with fibrous valvular deformity.

In *Hunter's syndrome* the clinical manifestations are similar, but deafness is more common. In *San Fillipo syndrome* mental retardation is more obvious. Skeletal changes are less and only hepartin sulphate is elevated in urine. In *Scheie's syndrome* there is no mental retardation and only chondroitin sulphate is present in excess in the urine. In *Morquio Brailsford disease* skeletal abnormalities are particularly prominent. The knees and elbows show limitation of movement whereas in contrast the fingers and wrists show ligamentous laxity. Epiphyseal dysplasia and osteoporosis are prominent radiologically and the urinary keratosulphate concentration is elevated.

Familial Mediterranean fever

This disease inherited in an autosomal recessive manner and

is almost confined to Ashkanazy Jews. Onset is usually in childhood and there is recurrent fever, abdominal pain and a symmetrical polyarthritis of large joints, each episode lasting only a few days. Synovial membrane biopsy and synovial fluid findings are those of an acute non-specific synovitis and joint destruction does not occur.

The serum α_2 and fibrinogen levels are markedly elevated the serum aetiocholanolone concentration may be raised and there is a slight increase in gammaglobulins. Amyloidosis of the perireticulin distribution is common and the relationship between amyloid formation and the protein abnormalities is of interest to those studying the pathogenesis of amyloidosis.

Hyperbetalipoproteinaemia

This disorder of lipoprotein metabolism is inherited in an autosomal recessive manner, and is characterized by tuberous, tendinous and periosteal xanthomatosis, xanthelasma palpebrarum, arcus, and the early occurrence of atherosclerotic heart disease, which may result in myocardial infarction. The biochemical hallmarks are elevation of β lipoproteins of ultracentrifuge density 1.019 to 1.063; cholesterol and phospholipid values are also increased; there is no plasma chylomicron opalescence and serum triglyceride levels are normal. Only homozygotes develop the disease but in heterozygotes the serum biochemical abnormalities are present, to a less marked degree. Apart from tendinous xanthomata, there may be a migratory polyarthritis of large joints in homozygotes which may be extremely acute, but which is usually nondestructive. Treatment is that of the disease, namely diet and clofibrate. The arthritis and heart disease are treated symptomatically.

Hyperuricaemia and gouty arthritis may occur in types III, IV and V hyperlipoproteinaemia.

Von Gierke's disease (type 1 glycogen storage disease)

The autosomal recessively inherited deficiency of glucose-6-phosphatase results clinically in hepatomegaly, failure to thrive, and convulsions. Death usually occurs in childhood. Biochemically there is hypoglycaemia particularly on withholding food, failure to respond with a rise in blood sugar following adrenaline, and an increased amount of normally structured liver glycogen. Due to a combination of an increased *de novo* rate of purine synthesis and a reduction in renal secretion of uric acid hyperuricaemia occurs and acute gouty arthritis has been reported.

Chapter 15

MISCELLANEOUS LOCOMOTOR SYSTEM DERANGEMENTS

NON-FAMILIAL CONDITIONS

Polymyalgia rheumatica

This disease is more common than ankylosing spondylitis or gout and diagnosis is important since effective treatment is available.

Onset is in the late sixties and is acute, with marked stiffness and pain in the shoulder girdle and neck which is usually worse in the morning. Females are more commonly affected than males. Constitutional symptoms may be marked and include fatigue, anorexia, weight loss and fever. The peri-articular tissues are affected more severely than muscles or synovium, although there may be swelling of the small joints of the hands, and knee effusions. Polymyalgia rheumatica is not a dumping ground for inconvenient clinical presentations but should be considered as a distinct clinical syndrome characterized by features most of which must be present before the clinical diagnosis is made.

It is particularly important to examine the eyes carefully. Sudden occlusion of the ophthalmic arteries with irreversible blindness is the major complication of the disease and is due to arteritis. Other vessels may be affected, particularly the temporal arteries, and, indeed, in one third of cases the disease evolves to a stage which is identical to that of temporal arteritis. A great deal more information is required before the interrelationships of these diseases can be understood. Scalp tenderness and loss of pulsation in the temporal arteries are useful diagnostic clues, but in any case of doubt it is essential to biopsy these vessels.

There may be a normochromic normocytic anaemia and hyperglobulinaemia, but the most obvious laboratory feature is a greatly elevated erythrocyte sedimentation rate. Electromyography, muscle enzyme and muscle biopsy findings are normal. Treatment of the vasculitis is with high dose corticosteroid therapy which may indeed be 'sight-saving'. Dramatic response to high dose *short term* corticosteroids is so frequent that failure to respond should raise doubts as to the initial diagnosis.

Fibrositis

This is a layman's term for any pain in the musculo-skeletal system. The complaint is extremely common and is of major economic importance to the country. Temperature, trauma, temperament and toxicity have been mooted as precipitating factors. No serious attempt has yet been made to subclassify the complaint and pathological studies are few and unhelpful. Until more attention is paid to this field it is impossible to construct any aetiological or pathogenetic basis for fibrositis. Clinically it is important to exclude any underlying characterizable musculo-skeletal disorder or general medical disease such as hypo-thyroidism. A personality disorder may be present. Management can only be symptomatic, but response to anti-inflammatory and anagesic drugs is often poor.

Tietze's syndrome

This comprises recurrent chest pain accompanied by fusiform swelling of the costochondral joints. The pain may be localized or may radiate mimicking pleurisy, angina, intercostal neuritis or leukaemia. Histologically peri-articular soft tissue inflammatory changes are seen, but the cartilage is normal. The syndrome occurs most frequently in young adults.

Stiff man syndrome

This rare disease of the elderly is characterized by symmetrical proximal muscle stiffness, the patient assuming the 'guardsman-like' stance and gait. Tonic spasms may occur. The muscles are firm on palpation and the reflexes are normal. Electromyography shows the pattern of continuous voluntary movement and the differential diagnosis includes chronic tetanus. Aetiology is un-known, but treatment with chlordiazepoxide or diazepam may be beneficial.

The painful shoulder

This is a very common complaint and, in addition to arthritis of the joint, may be due to one of several local syndromes.

Rotator cuff syndrome

Calcific deposits in the tendons of supraspinatus, infraspinatus, teres minor or subscapularis may produce pain and dysfunction. Limitation of movement and pain are most marked from 70° to 130° of abduction. Rupture of these calcific deposits into the subdeltoid bursa may cause acute exacerbations. Tendon rupture or frozen shoulder may occur.

Rupture of the supraspinatus tendon, occurring for example with a fall on the outstretched hand, is usually easily diagnosed since this muscle subserves the beginning of abduction.

Bicipital tendinitis

A synovitis of the long head of biceps in the bicipital groove on the lateral aspect of the humerus produces local pain and pain on external rotation. Treatment can be very difficult, but a local corticosteroid injection may help. Transposition of the tendon from the groove may be necessary.

Frozen shoulder

This may follow either of the above syndromes, may occur *de novo*, or may complicate local trauma, operation, myocardial infarction, tuberculosis, cerebrovascular accidents or cervical cord or disc disease. This is a disease of the elderly which is insidious in onset. The patient complains of pain which may radiate down the arm, and severe stiffness. Although it may last over a year complete resolution usually occurs even without treatment. Local heat, exercise and local injection of corticosteroids are usually prescribed with varying lack of success.

Shoulder hand syndrome

In this syndrome, which also occurs in the elderly, to the clinical manifestations of the frozen shoulder, are added pain, stiffness, swelling and trophic changes in the hand. Muscle

161

wasting and contractures follow, and skin atrophy and even thickening may simulate scleroderma. Radiologically, severe local osteoporosis may be seen. The aetiology is unknown, but the syndrome commonly follows local injury or sepsis, cervical cord or disc disease, cerebrovascular accident or myocardial infarction. Recently a relationship to isoniazid has been postulated. In many instances, however, no precipitant is discernable. Treatment is unsatisfactory but heat, exercises and even stellate ganglion block have been claimed to be effective. In many patients inexorable progression to crippling joint deformities occurs despite all intervention. Intra-articular corticosteroids may be prescribed.

Tennis elbow

Pain is localized at the lateral humeral epicondyle and there may be local signs of inflammation. Trauma is usually invoked to explain the pain. The syndrome is self-limiting, but may be relieved by local injection of corticosteroids.

Painful heel

Pain in the heel may be due to a *stress fracture* of the calcaneum which usually occurs in young soldiers and which may not be apparent radiologically for 2 weeks. It may also be due to a *plantar fasciitis* which occurs *de novo* particularly in the elderly, or may accompany diseases such as ankylosing spondylitis, Reiter's disease, rheumatoid arthritis or gonococcal infection.

Painful forefoot

Localized pain in the forefoot may have several causes. A *plantar digital neuroma* causes severe lancinating pain which may radiate into the toe or up the leg. Local tenderness will be elicited between the first and second metatarsal heads. Operative removal is indicated. In the *March fracture*, which is a stress fracture of a metatarsal produced by marching, pain and tenderness are localized to the bone and the history provides the diagnosis. *Kohler's disease* is osteochondritis of the second metatarsal head. The foot is swollen, the intrinsic muscles are atrophied and plantar flexion and claw foot follow. Radiologically the metatarsal head is broad and flattened with a reduction in bone density. Treatment is with a metatarsal bar and exercise. Pain in the forefoot may also be produced by *arthritis* or by stretching of the metatarsal ligaments.

Carpal tunnel syndrome

This is an entrapment neuropathy of the median nerve underneath the flexor retinaculum in the carpal tunnel. It is particularly common in females. There is wasting of the thenar eminence with weakness, particularly of the abductor pollicis brevis muscle. Paraesthesia and anaesthesia occur in the skin supplied by the median nerve and may be most marked at night or after exercise. The distribution may not be 'classical', but the fifth finger is always spared. Parathesia may be provoked by tapping or by pressure over the carpal tunnel (Tinel's sign). Prolongation of motor conduction time may be detected by electromyography. Diagnosis may be complicated by radiation of pain up the forearm.

Treatment is by surgical decompression. At operation thickening and fibrosis of the synovium of the flexor tendon sheaths is usually seen and this may be of unknown aetiology or may be the result of rheumatoid arthritis, systemic lupus erythematosus or scleroderma. The syndrome may also be caused by local benign neoplasms, pregnancy, myxoedema, amyloid, myeloma, haemophilia or gout.

Cervico-brachial syndrome

Elements of the brachial plexus may be compressed at the thoracic outlet either by soft tissues, for example, in the scalenus anticus syndrome, or by bone in the case of a cervical rib or an abnormal first thoracic rib. Onset is usually in the fifth decade and the greater frequency of symptoms in females is said to be related to the carrying of heavy shopping bags. Clinically there is pain, paraesthesia or anaesthesia and muscle wasting or weakness usually in the distribution of C7 and T1 (Fig. 9). The pain is dull and boring in character and may be most severe in the evening. Angina may be simulated. Vasomotor symptoms, Raynaud's phenomenon, unequal radial pulses and, rarely, arterial thrombosis may be present. Diagnosis is from other

163

causes of pain in the shoulder, from neurological causes of wasting of the hand muscles including ulnar and median neuropathies, carpal tunnel syndrome, motor neurone disease, multiple sclerosis, spinal cord neoplasm syringomyelia and cervical spondylosis, and from other causes of Raynaud's phenomenon. Treatment is surgical if the symptoms are severe.

Reticulohistiocytosis

This rare disease of unknown aetiology is a granuloma of skin, mucous membranes and synovium. Females are affected more commonly than males and large purple nodules develop in the skin over bony prominences, tendons and joints. Large multinucleated giant cells with glycolipid-laden cytoplasm are seen. A destructive rheumatoid-like arthritis may occur which may be as severe as arthritis mutilans, but serological tests for rheumatoid factor are negative. An abnormal circulating lipoprotein may be detected. Clinically nodules at the elbows and over tendons co-existing with arthritis may also occur in rheumatoid arthritis, gout, agammaglobulinaemia, Still's disease, granuloma annulare and hyperbetalipoproteinaemia.

Relapsing polychondritis

This exceptionally rare disease of unknown aetiology is characterized by recurrent painful inflammation of the cartilage of the ear, nose, larynx and joints, associated with fever. On occasions the urinary glycosaminoglycan concentration may be elevated.

Pigmented villonodular synovitis

This exceptionally rare disease most commonly affects the knee joints. Clinically there is marked synovial hypertrophy and histologically large numbers of polyhedral stromal cells, cellular infiltration, haemosiderin-laden macrophages and villous hypertrophy are seen. The aetiology of this disease is unknown, but some authorities consider that it may predispose to malignancy. Clinical suspicion is usually raised by the repeated aspiration of blood stained synovial fluid.

Synovial tumour

These are exceptionally rare and occur in young adults. Clinically they present as painless swellings and metastasize rapidly. Limb amputation or wide local excision and radiotherapy may give a 50 per cent 5 year survival rate. It is interesting that malignant change is so uncommon in a tissue which is so frequently the seat of intense proliferative reactions.

Ollier's disease (enchondromatosis)

This rare non-familial developmental defect of cartilage is manifest clinically as centrally placed nodular masses especially in the metacarpals and phalanges of the fingers, which may undergo malignant degeneration. The pathogenesis is thought to be proliferation from ectopic cartilage cell nests. In association with cavernous haemangiomata and subcutaneous phleboliths the eponymous title Maffucci's syndrome is applied.

Arthrogryposis multiplex congenita

This rare congenital disorder is essentially a descriptive term for severe joint flexion contractures of unknown aetiology which may be associated with absent patellae, micrognathia, cardiovascular lesions, and neuro muscular diseases.

Acro-osteolysis (disappearing bone disease)

This may occur without any known cause or may be associated with trauma, haemangiomata, scleroderma, hyperparathyroidism, psoriatic arthritis, or rheumatoid arthritis. An inherited generalized symmetrical acro-osteolysis of unknown aetiology, particularly affecting bones of feet, wrists and elbows, may occur in association with other skeletal deformities and with renal impairment.

FAMILIAL

Achondroplasia

This disease is transmitted by an autosomal dominant gene. The defect is of cartilage ossification and is confined to the skull and long bones. The trunk is normal, the head large and the limbs short. The hands are squat with fingers of equal length ('trident hand'), the epiphyses are large and the diaphyses short.

Angiokeratoma corporis diffusa (Fabry's disease)

This rare sex-linked recessive enzyme defect is characterized by periodic fever and arthralgia, telangiectasis, corneal dystrophy and renal disease. Glycolipid inclusion bodies are found in skin and renal cells and this disease may be related to the mucopolysaccharidoses.

Osteogenesis imperfecta

This is a rare disease which is transmitted by an autosomal dominant gene. Clinically there is severe osteoporosis with multiple fractures which may even occur *in utero*, blue sclerae, ligamentous laxity and thinning of the skin. Otosclerotic deafness may occur in later life.

Nail patella syndrome

The main interest in this rare disease was provided by the demonstration of genetic linkage between the responsible autosomal dominant gene, and the gene loci for the ABO blood group system.

Clinically there is deformity of the nails, hypoplasia or absence of the patella and hypoplasia of the radial head and scapula. Iliac horns are seen on X-ray.

Hereditary multiple exostoses (diaphysial aclasia)

Multiple cartilage capped exostoses which may be premalignant develop around the shoulder and pelvic girdles, the knee and ankle joint. The genetic mechanism has not yet been elucidated.

Chapter 16

DRUGS USED IN THE TREATMENT OF THE CHRONIC ARTHRITIDES

Most of the chronic arthritides are still incurable diseases and their management must therefore include the use of non-specific suppressive agents. It is particularly important in these circumstances to balance carefully the likelihood of therapeutic effect against the possibility of deleterious effect.

Aspirin (Fig. 37)

On the grounds of both efficacy and safety aspirin remains the drug of choice in the management of most of the chronic arthritides. The dose of aspirin must be in excess of 3 g per day to achieve anti-inflammatory effect. The method of action of salicylates is unknown. They have been shown, experimentally, to antagonise the effect of kinins, of 5-hydroxytryptamine and of slow reacting substance (SRS). They stabilize the lysosomal membrane, uncouple oxidative phosphorylation and interact with the prostaglandins. Thus they may affect the inflammatory response at many different points. Aspirin (acetylsalicylic acid) and the salicylate ion (Fig. 37) behave differently in pharma-

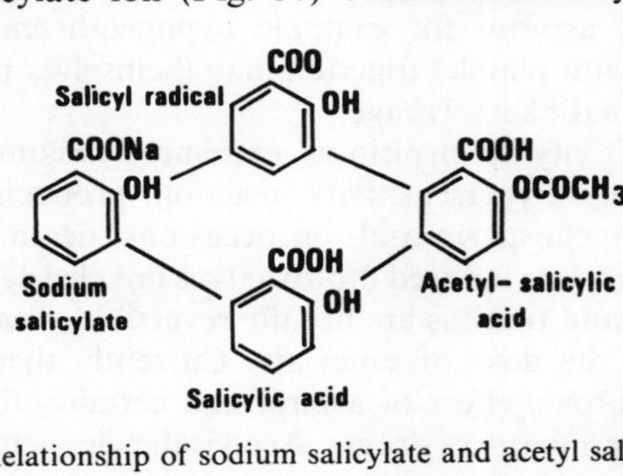

Fig. 37 Relationship of sodium salicylate and acetyl salicylic acid.

Recently a great deal of attention has been focused upon side effects of salicylates. The most common side effect is minor gastro-intestinal upset and dyspepsia which may be reduced by giving salicylates in the form of aloxiprin (Palaprin) which is a combination of aluminium oxide and aspirin, or enteric coated salicylate (Entrosalyl). It is important to remember, that 70 per cent of patients with arthritis will tolerate anti-inflammatory doses of salicylates when these are properly prescribed.

Over three quarters of patients taking aspirin lose a small amount of blood in the stool each day. The amount is usually less than 5 ml and only rarely does this give rise to iron deficiency anaemia. Indeed, the beneficial effect of salicylates on rheumatoid arthritis itself outweighs this disadvantage. The validity of this statement is borne out by the fact that patients with rheumatoid arthritis who respond to salicylates demonstrate not a fall, but a rise in haemoglobin levels over a period of years. On occasions aspirin may provoke moderate or even massive gastro-intestinal haemorrhage. It is probable, however, that aspirin is only one of the factors involved and that this only occurs in patients who are otherwise predisposed to this, for example, by pre-existing hypovitaminosis C. Furthermore, the frequency of gastro-intestinal haemorrhage must be viewed against the enormous number of aspirin tablets which are ingested each year. The risk is undoubtedly extremely small. Interestingly, it has been shown that patients who have previously suffered from salicylate induced gastro-intestinal haemorrhage showed no significant increase in faecal blood loss compared with control subjects when they were re-exposed to salicylates at a later period. The mechanism of gastro-intestinal haemorrhage is not entirely clear, although it seems likely that the effect is a local one. Other properties of aspirin, for example hypoprothrombinaemia or interference with platelet function may themselves predispose to gastro-intestinal haemorrhage.

Hypersensitivity to aspirin is extremely uncommon and is similar to any hypersensitivity reaction producing localized urticaria, bronchospasm and, on occasions, death. The pathogenesis or salicylate induced ototoxicity is not clearly understood, but deafness and tinnitus are usually reversible, disappearing on reduction of the dose of salicylate. Currently there is interest in the nephrotoxic effect of aspirin and certain other analgesic and anti-inflammatory drugs. Acetylsalicylic acid causes an increase in urinary renal cell count. The mechanism of this effect is not understood. Whether aspirin either alone, or in combination with phenacetin paracetamol or codeine, may be implicated in the development of 'analgesic nephropathy' has not yet been determined. The possibility, however, should be constantly remembered and a close surveillance of urinary function is indicated in all patients receiving long term salicylate therapy.

Aspirin overdose is a particular hazard in children since the difference between a therapeutic and a toxic dose is small. The effects of salicylate poisoning are profound and their pathogenesis is complex.

In the first place there is a tendency to a metabolic acidosis. Increased basal metabolic rate and pyrexia, interference with the actions of dehydrogenases and transaminases enzymes, and dehydration all contribute to this.

In the second place there is a tendency to the development of a respiratory alkalosis produced by stimulation of the respiratory centre. Initially the tendency for blood pH to rise is combated by the kidney. Reabsorption of bicarbonate is reduced and an alkaline urine is secreted. There is a resultant loss of cations and water, and the serum bicarbonate falls.

The balance of these effects in an individual patient depends on many factors including age of the patient, the dose ingested, and the duration of poisoning.

In severe poisoning there may also be hypocalcaemia, hypoglycaemia and hypoprothrombinaemia. If the serum salicylate concentration exceeds 70 mg/100 ml the prognosis is poor.

Management of salicylate poisoning is determined to a large extent by the biochemical results and requires the closest collaboration between the biochemist and the clinician. Correction of dehydration is of prime importance. In severe cases renal dialysis should be considered.

Indomethacin

Indomethacin (Indocid) is an indole derivative which possesses potent anti-inflammatory effects. The initial reports of this drug were bedevilled by its introduction to medical practice at excessive dose levels and by inadequately controlled clinical assessments. The compound is of value in the management of patients with rheumatoid arthritis and other chronic arthritides and it can be considered to be roughly equi-potent with aspirin. The dose is approximately 100 to 150 mg per day, but the method of administration is of prime importance. Treatment should commence with a low dose (e.g. 25 mg b.d.) and the dose should be gradually increased until the maximum therapeutic effect has been obtained. Prescribed in this way the incidence and severity of side effects, which were widely reported in the earlier literature, may be greatly diminished. A 100 mg suppository formulation is available but although the frequency of dyspepsia may be reduced in this way, rectal irritation and bleeding limit its usefulness.

Approximately 10 to 20 per cent of patients taking this drug will develop headaches, dizziness or gastro-intestinal disturbance. Peptic ulceration with haematemisis or perforation may occur and a feature of indomethacin induced gastric ulcers is their large size. Skin rashes and fluid retention are uncommon.

Phenylbutazone

This is a pyrazolone derivative (Fig. 38), and is a highly effective anti-inflammatory analgesic drug. It is a potent hepatic microsomal enzyme inducer and will reduce the half life both of itself and of drugs similarly metabolized such as phenobarbitone. Phenylbutazone is highly but loosely bound to plasma proteins and will displace other compounds which are also protein bound. This results in potentiation of anticoagulant, sulphonamide, and biguanide effects and also in retardation of excretion of phenylbutazone. The blood levels of phenylbutazone represent a

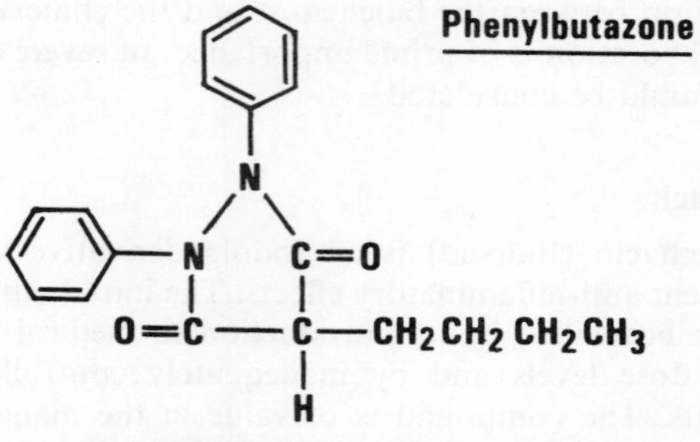

Phenylbutazone

Fig. 38 Structure of phenylbutozone.

170

balance between the excretion and metabolism of the drug, the net effect being cumulative.

The list of toxic effects is formidable, and includes anorexia, nausea, vomiting, dyspepsia, xerostomia, stomatitis and diarrhoea. Febrile reactions with lymphadenopathy and a variety of allergic skin rashes or even the Stevens-Johnson syndrome may occur. Liver or renal damage may result from its use, and peptic ulceration may develop and be complicated by haemorrhage or perforation. Goitre due to an organification block may occur. Weight gain due to salt and water retention may precipitate congestive cardiac failure in patients with hypertension or heart disease.

By far the most serious toxic hazards are agranulocytosis and aplastic anaemia. Leucopenia, and thrombocytopenia may also occur. Agranulocytosis occurs in young patients soon after commencing treatment whereas aplastic anaemia occurs in the elderly and may commence after many months of treatment. However, the incidence of blood dyscrasias is low and has been estimated as occurring once in every 150,000 'patient-months' of treatment.

Despite this list of side effects phenylbutazone, given in a dose of less than 300 mg per day, is a useful drug, when other analgesic and anti-inflammatory drugs have failed. There is no evidence that other derivatives of phenylbutazone, such as oxyphanbutazone, offer any advantage.

Ibuprofen and the fenemates

These recently introduced compounds have been shown to have analgesic and anti-inflammatory effects. Ibuprofen is one of a series of phenylalkanoic acid derivatives. The drug is less effective than aspirin, but possesses the advantage of a low incidence of side effects. In particular gastro-intestinal upset is uncommon. The recommended dose is 400 mg three times a day by mouth. The fenemates, mefenamic and flufenamic acids are two anthranilic acid derivatives which have recently been introduced as antirheumatic agents. These drugs are less effective than aspirin, and nausea, dyspepsia and diarrhoea are their main disadvantages. Potentiation of coumarin anticoagulants, transient leucopenia, and haemolytic anaemia have also been reported. The dose of mefenamic acid is 250 to 500 mg by mouth four times a day and flufenamic acid 200 mg three times a day by mouth.

ANALGESICS

Phenacetin

Phenacetin is a para-aminophenol derivative which has mild analgesic, but no anti-inflammatory properties. As such it is unsuitable on its own in the treatment of patients with rheumatoid arthritis. Acute or chronic haemolytic anaemia, macrocytic anaemia, pancytopenia, methaemoglobinaemia and sulphaemoglobinaemia, and jaundice may occur with phenacetin therapy.

The main concern at the present time is with the drug's nephrotoxicity. Renal papillary necrosis and interstitial nephritis have been reported in patients who have received phenacetin. However, these patients have also received other analgesics, including codeine, paracetamol and aspirin, and at the present time it is not possible to incriminate any single drug in the pathogenesis of this disease, which is now referred to as analgesic nephropathy. Although the precise incidence of analgesic nephropathy is not yet known, the disease is probably common and contributes something like 10 per cent to the pool of patients requiring chronic renal dialysis. Of all causes of chronic renal failure, it may be one with the best prognosis since strict avoidance of all analgesics seems to result in regression. It is therefore important to diagnose this disease. There is some evidence to suggest that a high fluid intake may have prophylactic value.

Because of the possible renal complications phenacetin has been removed from many analgesic mixtures and proprietary preparations, although it is still included in Tab. Codeine Co. B.P. There seems little justification for the use of this weak and potentially toxic analgesic in the management of an essentially inflammatory disease.

Paracetamol

Paracetamol is formed in the liver as the principal metabolite of phenacetin. The drug is a useful analgesic, but lacks anti-inflammatory properties and can only be used as an adjunct to anti-inflammatory therapy. The dose recommended is 1 to 2 g four times a day. Massive overdosage may cause liver necrosis and hypoglycaemia.

Codeine

Codeine, a weak analgesic, is usually combined with other

compounds. The drug has mild addictive properties, and often causes constipation, and is not therefore suitable alone in the management of rheumatoid arthritis.

Dihydrocodeine

Dihydrocodeine, although popular at present, offers no real advantage over codeine. Constipation is commonly induced. It is mildly addictive and may produce respiratory depression in overdosage.

Pentazocine and dextropropoxyphene

These newly introduced analgesic drugs have no anti-inflammatory properties and should not be employed alone in the treatment of the inflammatory arthritides. They may produce dyspepsia, and have central side effects but are not at present thought to be addictive.

Crysotherapy

Gold injections have been shown to be effective in rheumatoid arthritis.

It is customary to administer a test dose of 10 mg of sodium aurothiomalate, and to follow this with 20 mg the next week and 50 mg for succeeding weeks until 1 g has been given. The injections are given intramuscularly following urinalysis, examination of the skin, and performance of a full blood examination. The onset of therapeutic effect is delayed and may not be apparent for up to 3 months, but if no response has been obtained in 4 to 5 months treatment should be discontinued. Clinical effect is accompanied by a fall in the titre of rheumatoid factor, gold and chloroquine being the only drugs with this action. If a remission is obtained gold should be continued at a lower dose level thereafter, and should not be prescribed in 'courses'. It is not true that patients suffering toxic effects respond better to gold, as was previously suspected. Gold should never be given before an *adequate* trial of conservative measures and aspirin, and, when prescribed, meticulous follow up of patients is mandatory. The frequency and severity of side effects of gold unfortunately militate against its widespread use in the treatment of rheumatoid arthritis.

Gold is particularly toxic to skin and mucous membranes, the kidney, liver and bone marrow. Stomatitis, gastro-enteritis, exfoliative dermatitis, proteinuria and haematuria due to membranous glomerulonephritis, jaundice, peripheral neuropathy and alopecia may occur. The most serious complications, however, are leucopenia, thrombocytopenia, aplastic anaemia and agranulocytosis, all of which may be fatal. Side effects, and indeed also therapeutic effects, are to some extent dose related. However, there is such variation between the metabolism and excretion of gold in individual patients as measured by the usual methods, that it is extremely difficult to predict toxicity from the serum, urine or even tissue gold levels. More accurate methods of estimation recently introduced offer hope of overcoming this problem. Mild proteinuria alone does not demand the cessation of gold therapy, but pruritis and eosinophilia may predict the occurrence of a hypersensitivity reaction.

The mode of action of gold is not yet known. Interference with —SH group reactions, lysosomal membrane stabilization and interference with lymphocyte function have all been demonstrated, but their individual or collective relevance to the therapeutic effect has not been established.

Chloroquine and hydroxychloroquine

These drugs have been shown to have a beneficial effect in rheumatoid arthritis. The compound most commonly prescribed is chloroquine in a dose of less than 300 mg per day. The effect is gradual and is associated with a fall in titre of rheumatoid factor. Toxic manifestations include skin rashes, gastro-intestinal upsets, leucopenia, neuromyopathy, and alopecia.

The most serious side effect is blindness which results from accumulation of the drug in the pigment of the retina and which may be irreversible. It has been estimated that between 1 in 1000 and 1 in 2000 patients on long term therapy develop this complication. Interestingly the complication is confined to Caucasians. It seems that pigment elsewhere other than the retina protects the eye and that the retinopathy is an exaggerated local reflection of a generalized pigment disorder being associated with pigmentary changes in the skin, hair and eyelashes. The appearances on ophthalmoscopy are those of macular oedema surrounded by a pigmented circle with a peripheral depigmented zone, appearances often referred to as the 'bull's eye' fundus. Electro-oculograms and colour vision testing may be used in addition to standard clinical methods to detect early toxicity.

Retinopathy may progress even following withdrawal of the drug, but corneal deposits due to chloroquine, which are more common than retinopathy, disappear on withdrawal. Photosensitivity and increased porphyrin excretion may also be produced by chloroquine.

Although clinical benefit has been demonstrated in rheumatoid arthritis, the toxic effects of chloroquine and hydroxychlorine necessitate fastidious medical and ophthalmological supervision and reduce the potential value of these compounds. Antimalarial drugs do not have the usual anti-inflammatory effects in standard pharmacological test syptoms. Their mode of action may be related to their interactions with nucleoproteins, to stabilization of lysosomal membranes or to blockage of the sulphydryl/disulphide exchange reactions.

Corticosteroid therapy

Corticosteroids are undoubtedly the most powerful agents in the control of inflammation in rheumatoid arthritis although they probably do not affect the ultimate course of the disease. In view of their many side effects it is particularly important that they should be given only after other simple anti-inflammatory drugs have been given an adequate trial and found to be ineffective. The indications for corticosteroid therapy are discussed with the relevant diseases. Low dose corticosteroid therapy is too frequently instituted in severe disease on a long term basis. One of the least exploited and most useful methods of administration is the short term course of low dose prednisolone given to tide a patient over a temporary exacerbation in disease activity. Patients receiving long term treatment should be frequently re-assessed to determine the necessity of continued treatment.

Although there has been a great deal of controversy regarding the particular preparation which is best prescribed, there is no evidence that any newer drug is more effective or safe than prednisolone. In general the dose should be kept below 10 mg per day and treatment is best started with 2 mg b.d. orally. Over 10 to 15 mg/day the side effects become much more frequent and severe, and there is no evidence of greater clinical effect.

(Exceptions to this rule in systemic lupus erythematosus, dermatomyositis, polyarteritis nodosa and 'malignant' rheumatoid arthritis are described with these diseases.) One advantage of giving alternate day regimens is that the side effect of cerebrohypothalamopituitary adrenal (CHPA) axis suppression is probably less with this regimen, but control of symptoms may be sacrificed.

To understand the side effects of adrenal corticosteroids it is necessary to know their metabolic effects and the normal control of their secretion.

Cortisol is synthetized in and secreted from the adrenal cortex under the control of adrenocorticotrophic hormone (ACTH), which itself is controlled by corticotrophin releasing factor (CRF) produced in the hypothalamus. The entire system is influenced by the cerebral cortex (Fig. 39). Under normal conditions both ACTH and plasma cortisol release possess a circadian rhythm, the highest levels being reached at 8.00 a.m. and the lowest at midnight. ACTH release is controlled by the plasma cortisol in a 'negative feedback' fashion. The function of this physiological cerebrohypothalamo pituitary adrenal axis is to provide for, and to regulate, the increased levels of cortisol required in any stressful situation.

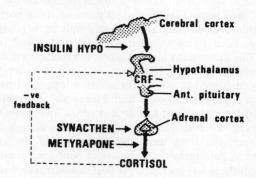

Fig. 39 Cerebro hypothalamo pituitary adrenal axis.

Briefly the metabolic effects of cortisol include increased gluconeogenesis with decreased peripheral glucose uptake which may result in glycosuria; increased protein catabolism with negative nitrogen balance; renal tubular retention of sodium and

176

water, and excretion of potassium; increased fat mobilization and deposition; uricosuria; increased calcium excretion and vitamin D antagonism. Their 'anti-inflammatory' effects are; reduced antibody production; impaired cell mediated immune response; reduction in lymphoid tissue and in circulating eosinophils and stabilization of lysosomes.

These effects may be considered generally as either 'glucocorticoid', 'mineralocorticoid', 'anti-inflammatory' or undetermined and explain the unwanted effects of corticosteroid therapy (Table 14).

Table 14 Corticosteroid side effects

Action		Effect
Stimulate gluconeo-genesis	N_2 excretion collagen loss	skin, muscle atrophy, purpura, osteoporosis
Glucocorticoid	Block insulin induced glucose transport across cell membrane	Hyperglycaemia, diabetes*
Mineralo-corticoid	Increase Na^+ reabsorption $\therefore$ H^+ and K^+ excretion	Oedema C.C.F. Hypertension* Hypokalaemia*
Anti-inflammatory	Reduce vascular permeability stabilize lysosomes, reduce leucocyte migration, reduce antibody titres,* reduce homograft rejection and tuber-culin reaction*	Masking*/ reactivation of infection (viral, TB, bacterial)
Not determined	Acne, hirsutism (? dehydro-epiandrosterone), peptic ulcer complications, psychosis,* cataract, glaucoma, avascular necrosis bone, fat redistribution (buffalo hump, moon face), myopathy, menstrual irregularity, increased calcium excretion and vitamin D antagonism	
Axis suppression		

* Especially in high dose.

177

Slight structural alterations may have a profound effect on the balance of these actions. For example fluorodination and hydroxylation causes less mineralocorticoid effect but seems to confer the property of inducing myopathy. With substitution of a methyl for the hydroxyl group at carbon 16 (Fig. 40) the mineralocorticoid effect is almost removed. A double bond at C_{1-2} enhances the glucocorticoid and reduces the mineralocorticoid effect.

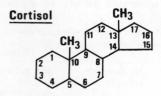

Fig. 40 Steroid nucleus.

Corticosteroids are largely conjugated by the liver although there are other degradative pathways. The clinical value of urinary derivatives of cortisol has been bedevilled by methodological and interpretative problems. More accurate assessment of adrenal status is afforded by radioisotopic determination of cortisol secretion rate, or by estimation of free 11 OH corticosteroids in blood or urine, but neither method is as yet routinely available. In practical terms. '11 OHCS' is measured in the routine laboratory by a simple fluorescent technique which is adequate for clinical purposes. This measures cortisol, corticosterone, cholesterol and some non-specific chromogens.

Dynamic tests of the C–H–P–A axis which are mostly widely used are the Synacthen test, the insulin hypoglycaemia test, the metyrapone test and the lysine vasopressin test. An adequate rise in 11 OHCS following the injection of synthetic adrenocorticotrophic hormone ('Synacthen', β 1–24 ACTH) guarantees integrity of the adrenal cortex although the higher centres may be abnormal. If an abnormal response is obtained and then confirmed by a prolonged synacthen test then the adrenal cortex is suppressed and the entire axis is unable to operate.

The most sensitive test for the integrity of the higher centres of the CHPA axis is an adequate rise of plasma cortisol in response to hypoglycaemia induced by insulin. The blood glucose must drop below 40 mg or the test is invalid. Plasma cortisol levels are measured $\frac{1}{2}$, 1, 1$\frac{1}{2}$ and 2 hours after insulin injection and the results are compared with responses obtained in a large number of normal controls. Hypoglycaemia probably acts at the level of the cerebral cortex thus testing the entire CHPA axis. Metyrapone, an 11 β hydroxylase inhibitor, blocks the synthesis of endogenous cortisol thus stimulating ACTH release, and is most useful in detecting hypopituitarism. A negative result is unreliable. The lysine vasopressin test is stressful and may induce angina or rarely even myocardial infarction. A preliminary electrocardiogram should be performed. Lysine vasopressin stimulates the hypothalamic part of the axis, but on occasions it probably also acts at a cortical level also. This test is being used less frequently now than formerly.

In rheumatological practice these tests are employed to test the integrity of the C–H–P–A axis in corticosteroid treated patients in whom the question of axis suppression arises. Axis suppression is a function of both the dose and the duration of treatment. There is less danger of suppression with doses of less than 10 mg for less than one year than if either dose or duration is increased. The danger of axis suppression is that these patients may develop adrenal failure under stress and thus require to be given exogenous corticosteroids in these situations. Infection or other intercurrent illness and surgery are the most frequent problems encountered and unless axis integrity is shown by a normal diurnal rhythm, synacthen test and insulin hypoglycaemic test it is a wise precaution to give supplementary hydrocortisone to all patients who are receiving or who have recently received long term corticosteroids. Patients receiving corticosteroids should carry with them a card stating the preparation and dose prescribed.

The other side effects of corticosteroids are shown in Table 13. Corticosteroids may cause and certainly activate peptic ulcers and 'silent' perforation, or haematemesis may occur. Skin bruising and osteoporosis tend to occur together. Posterior subcapsular cataracts are less common than increased intra-ocular pressure which occurs in one third of patients. There is some evidence that although increased intra-ocular pressure, elevation of blood pressure, and glycosuria occur frequently, glaucoma, established hypertension and diabetes only occur in predisposed patients. Moon face acne, hirsutes, buffalo hump, menstrual irregularity and dyspepsia are common, but are not in themselves of great importance. Mood disturbance is common, but rarely a frank psychosis may develop. Myopathy reflects the negative protein balance, and is more common with fluoridinated compounds. Oedema is common in rheumatoid arthritis, but corticosteroid treatment is only one of many possible pathogenetic mechanisms. Hypokalaemia which is clinically significant is not common with low doses of prednisolone. Avascular necrosis of bone and osteoporosis occur particularly commonly in corticosteroid treated patients. Growth retardation in children may be a major problem.

Activation or masking of latent septic viral or tuberculous infection is a product of the effect for which the treatment is prescribed, namely the anti-inflammatory effect of corticosteroids. The mechanism of this effect is not yet clear despite a great deal of experimental work. Vascular permeability is diminished, the lysosomal membrane is stabilized, mitochondrial ATPase activity is increased, leucocyte migration is reduced, antibody production is diminished and cell mediated immune responses are impaired. The effect of corticol on prostaglandin metabolism is under investigation at present. The dose required to produce many of these effects is greatly in excess of those given to patients however.

Corticotrophin

Natural and synthetic corticotrophin are potent suppressors of the clinical effects of inflammation although neither has yet been shown to influence the course of the disease. Acthar gel or Synacthen must be given intramuscularly. The former is prescribed in units (20/day) and the latter in mg (0.5 mg alternate days). Adrenocorticotrophic hormone has more potent mineralocorticoid actions than prednisolone so hypokalaemia, hypertension and oedema are more marked. ACTH stimulates androgenic as well as gluco- and mineralo-corticoid hormones therefore there is less osteoporosis, muscle wasting or bruising and more hirsutism and acne. Administration by the intramuscular route results in less dyspepsia or peptic ulceration. Melanin stimulating hormone is included in the amino-acid sequence of ACTH so pigmentation is common. One of the main advantages of ACTH is its much reduced suppressive effect upon the CHPA axis compared with prednisolone. The main disadvantage of ACTH is that it seems to be more difficult to obtain satisfactory long term control of the disease.

Immunosuppressive drugs and penicillamine

There is much interest at the present time in the use of azathioprine, cyclophosphamide and other immunosuppressive drugs. The rationale for the use of such drugs derives from the concept of rheumatoid arthritis as an 'auto immune disease'. If the perpetuation of the disease depends upon the response to continued antigenic stimulation then theoretically it should be possible to control the disease by suppressing that response. The immune response may be suppressed by corticosteroids, by antilymphocytic serum, by irradiation or by cytotoxic drugs. Cytotoxic drugs include folic acid antagonists, purine or pyrimidine analogues and alkylating agents. Folic acid antagonists (methotrexate) act by inhibiting the enzyme folic acid reductase which converts folic acid to tetrahydrofolic acid, a substance which is necessary for nucleic acid synthesis. Purine synthesis can be blocked by purine analogues (mercaptopurine, azathioprine), and pyrimidine synthesis by pyrimidine analogues (fluorouracil). The alkylating agents, nitrogen, mustards and cyclophosphamide, are cytotoxic agents. They replace nucleoprotein hydrogen atoms with an alkyl group thus damaging the cell.

Satisfactory clinical remission in rheumatoid arthritis with cyclophosphamide and azothiaprine has been obtained in a large number of uncontrolled studies, but in a controlled study azathioprine was found to be toxic and symptomatically ineffective. It is conceivable, however, that the dose employed was insufficient, the duration of treatment too short or the disease too far advanced in these patients. No final judgement can yet be made on the place of these drugs, but it is interesting that at the doses commonly employed, clinically these compounds have anti-inflammatory rather than 'immunosuppressive' effects. More recent long term studies with azathioprine (3 g/kg) in rheumatoid arthritis have shown encouraging results.

In a similar class is the use of the drug penicillamine. D-Penicillamine (dimethylcysteine) is a metabolite of penicillin which contains sulphydryl groups and these groups combine with, and inactivate, essential —SH enzymes. It also acts as a bond breaking agent and it is this effect which is of interest in rheumatology. It is now known that complement-fixing antigen–antibody complexes are involved in tissue destruction and the rationale for the use of penicillamine is that it may dissociate these complexes. Penicillamine is certainly toxic, however, and has not yet been shown to alter the course of rheumatoid arthritis.

Appendix 1

THE EYE IN ARTHRITIS

The eye is frequently involved in the course of many of the arthritides and may also be affected by drugs used in the treatment of arthritis.

The most frequent ocular complications encountered in rheumatological practice are shown in Fig. 42 together with their associated diseases. In Fig. 41 the principal clinical features of these ocular complications are summarized.

Scleritis is probably an extension of episcleritis. Although less common than episcleritis it carries a more grave prognosis. Scleromalacia perforans is a rheumatoid nodule located in the sclera and probably arises from a patch of scleritis.

In Still's disease the primary lesion is the iridocyclitis. From this, clumps of degenerate cellular material and white cells float across the aqueous humour of the anterior chamber to form

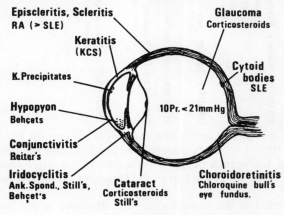

Fig. 41 The eye in arthritis. Clinical features.

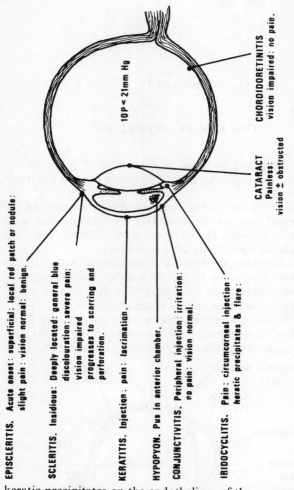

EPISCLERITIS. Acute onset : superficial : local red patch or nodule : slight pain : vision normal : benign.

SCLERITIS. Insidious : Deeply located : general blue discolouration : severe pain : vision impaired progresses to scarring and perforation.

KERATITIS. Injection : pain : lacrimation.

HYPOPYON. Pus in anterior chamber.

CONJUNCTIVITIS. Peripheral injection : irritation : no pain : vision normal.

IRIDOCYCLITIS. Pain : circumcorneal injection : keratic precipitates & flare :

IOP < 21mm Hg

CATARACT
Painless:
vision ± obstructed

CHOROIDORETINITIS.
vision impaired : no pain.

Fig. 42 The eye in arthritis. Signs of disease.

keratic precipitates on the endothelium of the cornea. The other ocular lesions of Still's disease are cataracts, and the development in the cornea of band keratopathy, the latter being an entirely separate process from the formation of keratic precipitates.

The other ocular complications are described in the relevant chapters.

184

Appendix 2

DIAGNOSTIC CRITERIA FOR RHEUMATOID ARTHRITIS

'Classical' Rheumatoid Arthritis

This diagnosis requires seven of the following criteria. In criteria 1 to 5 the joint signs or symptoms must be continuous for at least 6 weeks. (Any one of twenty features listed under 'Exclusions' will exclude a patient from this category.)

1. Morning stiffness.

2. Pain on motion or tenderness in at least one joint (observed by a physician).

3. Swelling (soft tissue thickening or fluid—not bony overgrowth alone) in at least one joint (observed by a physician).

4. Swelling (observed by a physician) of at least one other joint (any interval free of joint symptoms between the two joint involvements may not be more than 3 months).

5. Symmetrical joint swelling (observed by a physician) with simultaneous involvement of the same joint on both sides of the body (bilateral involvement of mid-phalangeal, metacarpophalangeal, or metatarsophalangeal joints is acceptable without absolute symmetry). Terminal phalangeal joint involvement will not satisfy the criterion.

6. Subcutaneous nodules (observed by a physician) overy bony prominences, on extensor surfaces, or in juxta-articular regions.

7. X-ray changes typical of rheumatoid arthritis (which must include at least bony decalcification localized to or greatest around the involved joints and not just degenerative changes)— degenerative changes do not exclude patients from any group classified as rheumatoid arthritis.

8. Positive agglutination test—demonstration of the 'rheumatoid factor' by any method that, in two laboratories, has been positive in not more than 5 per cent of normal controls; or positive streptococcal agglutination test.

9. Poor mucin precipitate from synovial fluid (with shreds and cloudy solution).

10. Characteristic histological changes in synovial membrane with three or more of the following: marked villous hypertrophy; proliferation of superficial synovial cells often with palisading; marked infiltration of chronic inflammatory cells (lymphocytes or plasma cells predominating) with tendency to form 'lymphoid nodules'; deposition of compact fibrin, either on surface or interstitially; foci of cell necrosis.

11. Characteristic histological changes in nodules showing granulomatous foci with central zones of cell necrosis, surrounded by proliferated fixed cells, and peripheral fibrosis and chronic inflammatory cell infiltration, predominantly perivascular.

When five criteria are present the diagnosis is 'definite' rheumatoid arthritis and when three criteria are present the term 'probable' rheumatoid arthritis is used.

INDEX